T0194572

LIVING OUTSIDE

THE LINES

It's Time to Discover the
Beauty in Being You!

YVONNE JONES

WESTBOW
PRESS®
A DIVISION OF THOMAS NELSON
& ZONDERVAN

Scripture quotations marked (NIV) are taken from the Holy Bible, New
International Version®, NIV®. Copyright © 1973, 1978, 1984, 2011 by Biblica,
Inc.™ Used by permission of Zondervan. All rights reserved worldwide. www.
zondervan.com The "NIV" and "New International Version" are trademarks
registered in the United States Patent and Trademark Office by Biblica, Inc.

Scripture taken from the King James Version of the Bible.

WestBow Press books may be ordered through booksellers or by contacting:

WestBow Press
A Division of Thomas Nelson & Zondervan
1663 Liberty Drive
Bloomington, IN 47403
www.westbowpress.com
1 (866) 928-1240

ISBN: 978-1-9736-4781-2 (sc)
ISBN: 978-1-9736-4782-9 (e)

Print information available on the last page.

WestBow Press rev. date: 02/15/2019

I dedicate this book to every beautiful woman in this world. Let us continue to grow and strengthen one another as we pursue Christ-like love and character.

To my Heavenly Father. Thank you for continually showing me how much you love me. All that I have ever done is because and through you. Your kind gentle words have given me daily strength to persevere past my fears and advance into the future that you have for me. There will never be enough words to express all that you are and continue to be. I offer everything that I do to glorify, honor, and praise your name now and forever.

I thank God for my loving Grandparents Jill and William Finnegan who have supported loved and cared for me through this journey. Your kindness and patience have never been forgotten or overlooked. I appreciate all that you have done and recognize how thoroughly blessed I am to have you in my life. Finally, I thank God for my parents Ronald and Elizabeth Jones. Although mine and my sibling's upbringing was not perfect, I am forever grateful to have been given parents that instilled the importance of a relationship with Christ into our lives. I am thankful to have grown up in a family surrounded by love and God. Although my relationship with Christ began many years later, I do believe that the fundamental truths laid in my heart were through my parents and other significant individuals involved in my upbringing.

Introduction

Thank you for taking with me this journey to a better understanding of yourself. Our days can become so hectic and busy that we forget to take the time to reflect and evaluate who we are, what we have been doing, and where we are going in life. Self-reflection needs to be done daily and in many different ways. Whether meeting a friend for coffee, going to church, talking to God and reading His Word, or perhaps writing out our feelings, addressing what we are going through is vital to improving our daily lives and the lives of those around us.

This book is my light to you. It is all of the lessons that I have learned over many years. God has brought me through so much and taught me a copious amount of lessons that apply to many women these days. This devotional is not meant to condemn or put anyone down but to encourage each one of us to reflect and see if, and where, we can improve. These devotions God and I have created are all about how we look at ourselves and the actions we take or do not take, because of these beliefs.

In many cases, we limit ourselves; we stifle who we were made to be and ultimately put ourselves in a box by believing there is only one way we should live. We become carbon copies of everyone else who, just like us, is trying to find fulfillment in the way we are told to. The title of this devotional says it all. As Christian women, it is unwise to follow after the ideas, beliefs, and morals this world has increasingly forced upon us, but rather step outside of these metaphorical lines and live in the standards that God has laid out for us. It can be difficult for each of us to understand who we are when the world is telling us who we should be. I want you to discover the beauty of being yourself, the beauty in who God created you to be, and the enormous amount of joy and freedom that goes along with it.

This month, we are going to cover some significant areas in which we can easily get caught up in. We will include our possessions, beauty, self-esteem, relationships, careers, and equality. As we go through these daily devotions, there will be questions for you to reflect on at the end of each one. I find it best to have a designated notebook to write down your answers, questions, and how you may be feeling throughout these four weeks. I am so excited to start this journey with you.

Possessions Day 1

Investing In Your Character

We all know the feeling; walking past those sparkling glass windows and seeing an outfit that looks as if it were made just for us. We stop, stare, and wonder just how much it will cost. We then peek behind the large mannequin to see aisles upon aisles of clothing that we've been eyeing online or while flipping through magazines. In many ways, it feels as if we need to add that new shirt to our ever-growing pile of clothes we wear once and are never seen again.

Materialistic items are funny like that. To us, we can never have enough. But to our lives, closets, wallets, and most importantly, God, we most certainly can. The ever-present anthem of the world today is the more, the merrier, the bigger, the better, etc. The problem with phrases like these is that they scream all or nothing. If you don't have everything or the latest of everything, then you don't have anything. If you don't have rows of shoes, closets about to burst, stacks of makeup, and the latest camera to capture all of it on, then you need an upgrade. Possessions can control how we think about ourselves and others. We are told they are a sign of wealth, beauty, and ultimately worth.

Let's look at a woman in the Bible who gave away the most valuable possession she had for something that was priceless.

Reading — Luke 7:36–-47 (NIV)

When one of the Pharisees invited Jesus to have dinner with him, He went to the Pharisee's house and reclined at the table. A woman in that town who lived a sinful life in that town learned that Jesus was eating at the Pharisee's house, so she came there with an alabaster jar of perfume. As she stood behind Him at his feet weeping, she began to wet his feet with her tears. Then she wiped them with her hair, kissed them, and poured perfume on them.

When the Pharisee who had invited him saw this, he said to himself, "If this man were a prophet, he would know who is touching him and what kind of woman she is—that she is a sinner."

Jesus answered him, "Simon, I have something to tell you." "Tell me, teacher," he said.

"Two people owed money to a certain moneylender. One owed him five hundred denarii, and the other fifty. Neither of them had the money to pay him back, so he forgave the debts of both. Now which of them will love him more?"

Simon replied, "I suppose the one who had the bigger debt forgiven." "You have judged correctly," Jesus said. Then he turned toward the woman and said to Simon, "Do you see this woman? I came into your house. You did not give me any water for my feet, but she wet my feet with her tears and wiped them with her hair. You did not give me a kiss, but this woman, from the time I entered, has not stopped kissing my feet. You did not put oil on my head, but she has poured perfume on my feet. Therefore, I tell you, her many sins have been forgiven—as her great love has shown. But whoever has been forgiven little, loves little."

Then Jesus said to her, "Your sins are forgiven."

This woman came to Jesus a sinner, like all of us. She did not have much to offer, but she brought one of the most expensive items she had: an alabaster box of perfume. This lady was cast down and ridiculed because she was a prostitute, but she laid down her possessions and herself at the feet of Jesus. She came humbly and willingly to Him with all she had, knowing that nothing could compare to the weight of sin. In Matthew 19:24 (NIV), Jesus said, "It is easier for a camel to go through the eye of a needle, than for someone who is rich to enter the Kingdom of God."

Why is this?

Jesus knew that those who believe they have everything and those who are more concerned about the accumulation of goods here on earth will never see the genuine need for a relationship with Him. Our heavenly Father truly wants a relationship with us, but we choose possessions, people, and sin over Him. Those who truly understand the sacrifice Jesus made for them on the cross and the perfect love He daily gives to us, will never have to be tricked or forced into a relationship with Christ. This woman had a deep understanding of who Jesus was and therefore offered the most precious item she had willingly. The perfume that she brought was worth a year's wages back then, and she humbly came to pour it on the feet of Jesus. Sacrificing our possessions is hard for many of us, including me. It is hard to give up what we want and in some cases need, but Jesus tells us in Matthew 8:36–37 (NIV),

"For what shall it profit a man if he shall gain the whole world and lose his soul? Or what shall a man give in return for his soul?"

In many cases, it is easy to fall into the trap of feeling like we *need* that new thing, whatever it may be. But it is crucial for us to remember where to place our priorities, and that is in Christ. This lady gave the best she had, and God gave her something money could not buy: forgiveness, relationship, and eternal life through Him. God provides us with a brand new experience in Him, and it isn't because we have the latest and greatest but through acceptance of Him and the sacrifice He made for us on the cross. This lady knew she had nothing left to lose. Her value was no longer placed on this world and what she had but on what she could have through Jesus. With women especially, advertisers and companies are always trying to sell us something. This can make it difficult for us to focus on our character. Instead, we focus more on keeping up with what everybody else has or the standards of this world that we feel obligated to uphold. When we begin to place importance on who we are rather than what we own, we truly discover how much more we have to offer than a perfect outfit.

Self-Reflection

- Do you feel the need to accumulate new things continuously, or can you be satisfied with what you have?
- What are you holding back from God today, and for what reason?
- How do you as an individual use what God has already given to you to better yourself and others financially, spiritually, and physically? How do you use the gifts and talents He has given you?
- How do you use what you have to bring honor to God and fulfill the purpose He has given you for your life?
- Where do you place your self-worth: in who you are or what you own?

Health Check ✓

- Does your physical appearance affect what you use or buy?
- In what ways do you use your money or time to conform to the way you are told to appear?

Takeaways

- You are more than what you own.
- God can't work with who you pretend to be. Be open, and give all you are to Him so that you can be transformed through Him.
- God doesn't need our money and possessions. His only desire is that we love Him the way He loves us and that we trust Him!
- Spend less time trying to live up to the impossible expectations this world has for you and more time in the presence of God, with whom you have already been, and will always be accepted and loved.
- Give more to your relationship with God—not only your money but your time too. He confirms just how amazing you are and all you can accomplish

Possessions Day 2

Leave Doubt and Grab Trust

Welcome back! I hope you're enjoying your journey so far of renewing your mind and body. Yesterday we spoke about remembering that our possessions do not define who we are or how much we are worth. We also touched briefly on using what God has already blessed us with to encourage and inspire others. Today we are going to continue on the topic of possessions by taking a look at a story about a widow.

So at this time God had sent a significant famine across the land, and there was barely any food anywhere! Elijah, a prophet of God's, was told to go to the land of Zarephath to find food and shelter from a woman until God broke the famine across the nation. I don't know about you, but I would be very skeptical to leave and travel into a foreign land to ask a woman that has never met me before, to give me her last bit of bread and water! When this woman met Elijah, and he told her his unusual request for food and shelter, he reassured her that God would provide for her and her son if she did so. The widow obeyed and gave him all she had. Although she was not sure how she would feed herself or her son, this woman decided to believe that God would provide for her needs. As we can see by the end of this passage, God not only gave her more than enough food but also saved the life of her only son. God says in his word:

Reading — 1 Kings 17: 7-24 (NIV)

Some time later the brook dried up because there had been no rain in the land. Then the word of the Lord came to him: "Go at once to Zarephath in the region of Sidon and stay there. I have directed a widow there to supply you with food." So he went to Zarephath. When he came to the town gate, a widow was there gathering sticks. He called to her and asked, "Would you bring me a little water in a jar so I may have a drink?" As she was going to get it, he called, "And bring me, please, a piece of bread."

"As surely as the Lord your God lives," she replied, "I don't have any bread—only a handful of flour in a jar and a little olive oil in a jug. I am gathering a few sticks to take home and make a meal for myself and my son, that we may eat it—and die."

Elijah said to her, "Don't be afraid. Go home and do as you have said. But first, make a small loaf of bread for me from what you have and bring it to me, and then make something for yourself and your son. For this is what the Lord, the God of Israel, says: 'The jar of flour will not be used up, and the jug of oil will not run dry until the day the Lord sends rain on the land.'"

She went away and did as Elijah had told her. So there was food every day for Elijah and for the woman and her family. For the jar of flour was not used up and the jug of oil did not run dry, in keeping with the word of the Lord spoken by Elijah.

Sometime later the son of the woman who owned the house became ill. He grew worse and worse and finally stopped breathing. She said to Elijah, "What do you have against me, man of God? Did you come to remind me of my sin and kill my son?"

"Give me your son," Elijah replied. He took him from her arms, carried him to the upper room where he was staying, and laid him on his bed. Then he cried out to the Lord, "Lord my God, have you brought tragedy even on this widow I am staying with, by causing her son to die?" Then he stretched himself out on the boy three times and cried out to the Lord, "Lord my God, let this boy's life return to him!" The Lord heard Elijah's cry, and the boy's life returned to him, and he lived. Elijah picked up the child and carried him down from the room into the house. He gave him to his mother and said, "Look, your son is alive!"

Then the woman said to Elijah, "Now I know that you are a man of God and that the word of the Lord from your mouth is the truth."

The Bible says:

"Faith is composed of what we hope for and is the evidence of things not seen."
Hebrews 11:1 (KJV)

To me, this passage reiterates this scripture. That we are to do and give what we can as God directs us, and in turn watch Him bless us more than we could ever imagine. One thing that I have come to understand when learning how to truly listen and obey God is that it is not always about just obeying, but also about HOW I obey. God loves a cheerful giver; he likes when you give fearlessly. Doubting when and how you will make it is not faith, but trusting God to provide for you and do what his Word says, is! This widow had no reason to believe Elijah, but she decided to put her fear aside and what could go wrong and put her trust in the almighty God. She trusted in the God who knows what each of us needs before we even need it and provides in advance. As women we have the built-in natural desire to care for others; some refer to this as "motherly nature." We feel responsible on some level for our family, relationships, homes, etc. I know one of the first questions I ask my younger siblings when checking up on them is: "have you eaten?" This is a silly example, but it is in our nature to make sure everyone is doing okay, so much so that we can begin to feel burdened or overwhelmed. We feel like we have to do everything and if we don't, nothing will get done. There's a song that says:

"Oh if he carried the weight of the world on his shoulders, I know he will carry you."

God doesn't need us to take responsibility for every situation, person, and circumstance that is in our lives. Our focus should be directed towards growing our faith so that we are able to lay our concerns at His feet, live in joy, and allow God to do what we simply cannot. Worry doesn't change the outcome, but doing all you can and trusting God to do what you can't, definitely does.

Self-Reflection

- What materialistic items do you feel stressed about not having enough of?
- Is this a NEED or a WANT? How do you know this?
- Have you been relying on yourself or God to provide for your everyday needs?
- HOW do you give? Cheerfully or with fear?
- What do the people in your life say about your spending? Is it positive or negative?
- Have you asked God about your spending?

Health Check ✓

- How do you think being worried and fearful is negatively impacting your health? (stress, high blood pressure, etc.)

Takeaways

- Don't stress! God has already taken care of the problem
- Even if you don't see or know exactly how something will work out, trust God!
- Don't let your fear cause you to make a bad choice
- Give fearlessly and with joy
- Refuse to operate out of doubt in your circumstances
- Make sure your need is actually a need, not based off what the world says you have to have

Possessions Day 3

Building Everlasting Treasure

Hey there! I hope that you're enjoying this week of devotions. We're going to continue with our topic of possessions and read a passage today that speaks about a rich man and a beggar.

Reading — Luke 16:19-31 (NIV)

"There was a rich man who was dressed in purple and fine linen and lived in luxury every day. At his gate was laid a beggar named Lazarus, covered with sores and longing to eat what fell from the rich man's table. Even the dogs came and licked his sores.

"The time came when the beggar died and the angels carried him to Abraham's side. The rich man also died and was buried. In Hell, where he was in torment, he looked up and saw Abraham far away, with Lazarus by his side. So he called to him, 'Father Abraham, have pity on me and send Lazarus to dip the tip of his finger in water and cool my tongue, because I am in agony in this fire.' But Abraham replied, 'Son, remember that in your lifetime you received your good things, while Lazarus received bad things, but now he is comforted here and you are in agony. And besides all this, between us and you a great chasm has been set in place so that those who want to go from here to you cannot, nor can anyone cross over from there to us.'

"He answered, 'Then I beg you, father, send Lazarus to my family, for I have five brothers. Let him warn them so that they will not also come to this place of torment.'

"Abraham replied, 'They have Moses and the Prophets; let them listen to them.' 'No, father Abraham,' he said, 'but if someone from the dead goes to them, they will repent.' "He said to him, 'If they do not listen to Moses and the Prophets, they will not be convinced even if someone rises from the dead.'

In the world today we are taught to look out for ourselves and to focus on our needs. We are seldom concerned about the struggles that others go through and this whether we recognize it or not, can demonstrate our selfish character. It's easy to get caught up everything going on in our lives. Sometimes we are so hyper-focused on ourselves, and what we want, we let our relationships with others fall apart; most importantly our relationship with God. Having a relationship with Christ allows our character to be transformed to reflect more of Him. When we reflect Christ, we will carry a loving and caring spirit towards others into each every relationship. The rich man in this story demonstrates the relationship that many of us have with Jesus and others nowadays. If we don't feel like we need the individual, then we just do not prioritize the relationship. If we do not think the individual adds to our lives, then it is not something that we want to pursue. The rich man had everything he could possibly want or desire on earth. He did not feel as if he needed to have a relationship with God because all his needs appeared to be met. Lazarus also was not of importance to his life in any way, so he paid no attention to his needs. As we can see Lazarus had nothing while on earth. He was weak, sick, and looked down upon, but after they had both died who ultimately had riches? The rich man had created a life built around wealth rather than eternal sustainability. Jesus did not tell this story to scare us into loving Him, but rather as a reminder to look past the cares and possessions of this world and realize there is life after death. That life that can be filled with so much more than the trinkets we hold so dear to us, and instead filled with so much peace, love, and freedom. Eternity is a lot longer than the years here on earth. We need to make sure that we are daily working on our eternal destiny. If we allow ourselves to really know Jesus; to love and obey Him, we can find joy in this life and into the next. Don't let the standards of this world be the focus of your life.

Self Reflection

- How giving are you?
- Are you hyper-focused on all of your needs or do you take time to listen and care for others?
- How do you show your love for others?
- Like the rich man in this story, do you only seek God in times of trouble?
- How can you become closer with God today?
- Lazarus was seen by the rich man daily, yet he never cared to help him. Is there anyone in your life that you see frequently that needs help? How can you make their life better?

Health Check ✓

- You've taken a significant step forward bettering your spiritual and mental health, how can you continue this and impact your physical health?

Takeaways

- People are more important than possessions; remember to strengthen them before you strengthen your materialistic wants

- God desires a deeper relationship with you. Seek him every day not just when you mess up
- Be concerned for others and show the love of Christ to everyone the way He shows it to you
- God has so much more for you than the treasures of this world. Ask Him to open your eyes to the life He destined you to live and the relationship He wants with you
- The riches of this world will fade, just like the titles, careers, and positions. Make sure you daily spend your time working on your eternity, not your present fleeting life

Possessions Day 4

All Want Is Not Greed, But All Gain Is Not Equal

Today our reading is a little lengthier than usual, but it is definitely worth the read. Jesus speaks on the topic of greed in the parable today. He warns against storing up goods for yourself and having more than one person could ever spend.

Reading — Luke 12:16-31 (NIV)

And he told them this parable: "The ground of a certain rich man yielded an abundant harvest. He thought to himself, 'What shall I do? I have no place to store my crops.'

"Then he said, 'This is what I'll do. I will tear down my barns and build bigger ones, and there I will store my surplus grain. And I'll say to myself, "You have plenty of grain laid up for many years. Take life easy; eat, drink and be merry."'

"But God said to him, 'You fool! This very night your life will be demanded from you. Then who will get what you have prepared for yourself?' "This is how it will be with whoever stores up things for themselves but is not rich toward God."

Then Jesus said to his disciples: "Therefore I tell you, do not worry about your life, what you will eat; or about your body, what you will wear. For life is more than food, and the body more than clothes. Consider the ravens: They do not sow or reap, they have no storeroom or barn; yet God feeds them. And how much more valuable you are than birds! Who of you by worrying can add a single hour to your life? Since you cannot do this very little thing, why do you worry about the rest? "Consider how the wild flowers grow. They do not labor or spin. Yet I tell you, not even Solomon in all his splendor was dressed like one of these. If that is how God clothes the grass of the field, which is here today, and tomorrow is thrown into the fire, how much more will he clothe you-you of little faith! And do not set your heart on what you will eat or drink; do not worry about it. For the pagan world runs after all such things, and your Father knows that you need them. But seek his kingdom, and these things will be given to you as well."

Greed is selfishness, which is the opposite of love and therefore the opposite of God. Sometimes we can feel as if we need to be selfish to get ahead and to have enough, but as read in the passage if God clothes the grass and feeds the crows how much more will He provide for us? God made us a little lower than the angels! He created us in HIS image and HIS likeness. He sent his only son to die for our sins so that we can live with him in paradise for eternity. God's love for us is indescribable and incomparable. We do not need to try and provide for ourselves, we do not have to try and work out our lives. Jesus goes on to tell us in verse 22-23 (NIV)

"Therefore I tell you, do not worry about your life, what you will eat; or about your body, what you will wear. For life is more than food, and the body more than clothes.

Jesus does not want us to be so concerned about how well we live life now that we forget that there is another life to come.

In verses 33 and 34 Jesus goes on to say, (NIV)

"Sell your possessions and give to the poor. Provide purses for yourselves that will not wear out, a treasure in Heaven that will never fail, where no thief comes near and no moth destroys. For where your treasure is, there your heart will be also."

Many times our hearts are in the treasures of this world. The desire to accumulate earthly riches drives what we do, how we speak, and how much we compromise to gain these. Jesus is reminding us that there is a greater treasure than what we can find here. We are called to live a life that is full of sacrifice and service to others. As we continue to live and do the will of our Father, we store everlasting treasure for ourselves in Heaven. Worldly goods are fleeting but Heavenly treasure will remain forever. Always remember however that a good deed does not mean you are a follower of Christ and does not mean that you are storing Heavenly treasures. God definitely wants us to be good people, but we will always fail to be so without Christ. The only way to eternal life in Heaven is through acknowledging Jesus Christ and the sacrifice He made for us on the cross. When we have faith in who Christ is and accept Him as our Lord and Saviour, we are now able to begin to build up our Heavenly treasures through a life that is rooted in obedience and love towards Him. We should meditate daily on the realization that God loves us and knows what is best. With this understanding rooted in our hearts, obeying and following what He has instructed us to do will not feel like an action we are doing begrudgingly, but instead as a wise decision to trust in our Heavenly Father.

Self Reflection

- Do you build up your earthly treasures or your Heavenly ones?

- Do you think that being a good person or doing good deeds makes you a Christian?
- Have you accepted Jesus as your Lord and Saviour? If not what is holding you back?
- What are some earthly treasures that you have been holding onto too tightly?
- What can you do today to build up your Heavenly wealth?
- Do you allow the pressures of this world to cause you to feel obligated to live a particular lifestyle?
- Do you allow your value to be based on how much you have or on who God says you are?

Health Check ✓

- Have you allowed what other people think you should look/have affect how you see yourself? (physically and mentally)

Takeaways

- Heavenly wealth cannot be bought like a lipstick. It is through a deep and real relationship with Christ
- We will never be good enough to receive the gifts God has for us; remember the mercy that God has had on each one of us and be thankful
- The blessings you will receive by doing what God has called you to do here on earth, is higher than anything you could ever own or buy
- The choices you make today will decide your blessings and where you will spend life eternally
- Keep your eyes focused on Heaven, not on this fading earth

If you have not accepted Jesus as your Lord and Saviour and want to do so, you can repeat this prayer below:

Lord Jesus, I need you. Thank you for dying on the cross to pay the price for my sins. Thank you for the gift of eternal life through your Son Jesus. I ask you to please forgive me of all my sins, and I receive you as my Lord and Saviour now and forever. Thank you, Jesus. Amen.

Possessions Day 5

Adding to or Devaluing Our Lives

We are five days into our first week of devotions on possessions and how they can control how we think and what we value. Today I want us to look at this topic from a different angle, and I want you to ask yourself this question:

What do the people around me invest in?

When the people you surround yourself with are on the same page as you, they act as a daily reminder to remain true to yourself. Values are important, they serve as a guide to the kind of person we want and chose to be. We don't always have the option to be around individuals that are the best for us, but we can ask God to show us who is beneficial and chose to be around them. Surround yourself with people that see more to life than how many zeros you have in your bank account. They will challenge you to dig deeper and see your worth. They will encourage you to see that your value goes beyond what you own and will help reveal just how irreplaceably unique God made you. One of the great things about a relationship with God is there is never a time that He will love you more than He does right now. Many of our relationships nowadays can be based on what you have to offer, how you look, what you have accomplished etc. These type of connections can reveal the way in which your inner circle begins to influence what is of value to you. It is essential to have people around you who strive to see you how God does and push you towards a life full of Him. For today's passage, I want us to look at some individual verses in the Bible regarding the importance of who we keep around us and how vital their values are. As we go through each one reflect on the people that are around you the most and if they steer you in the right direction.

Blessed is the one who does not walk not in the counsel of the ungodly, or stands in the way that sinners take, or sits in the seat of mockers

Psalm 1:1 (NIV)

The righteous choose their friends carefully but the way of the wicked leads them astray.

Proverbs 12:26

Walk with the wise and become wise, for a companion of fools suffers harm

Proverbs 13:20 (NIV)

Be not deceived: evil communications corrupt good manners

1 Corinthians 15:33 (KJV)

But actually, I wrote to you not to associate with anyone who claims to be a brother or sister but is sexually immoral, or covetous, or an idolater, or a slanderer, or a drunkard, or a swindler— Do not even eat with such people

1 Corinthians 5:11 (NIV)

Stay away from a fool, for you will not find knowledge on their lips

Proverbs 14:7 (NIV)

Now I urge you, brethren, to watch out for those who cause divisions and put obstacles in your way that are contrary to the teaching that you have learned. Keep away from them

Romans 16:17 (NIV)

As you read each one of these verses, did you reflect on the people that you've considered friends? Sometimes it is easy to see the good in your inner circle because you love them. It may be difficult to believe that their lifestyle choices or who they are may have an adverse effect or pull you towards becoming someone that you are not interested in being. Jesus calls us as Christians to live as an example to others of the life they could have through Christ. We cannot lead if we are following. We cannot testify to the freedom Christ has given us if we live in bondage to the way in which others want us to live. We need to make sure the people that we chose to be around are continually reminding of us of why we are here. We are not here for money, houses, fame and ultimately possessions. We are here to fulfill the calling that Jesus placed on us from the moment He breathed the breath of life into us. When we have individuals around us that are passionate about His calling, it will encourage us to live in the authentic and free life offered only through Jesus, therefore, helping us to lead others into the arms of our heavenly Father to experience this as well.

Self Reflection

- Do your friends push you towards the woman of God you are called to be?
- Do you have like-minded individuals around you?
- What do your close friends value or would say is most important to them? Is this what you value or want to as well?
- Are you influencing your friends or being affected by them? Is this benefiting you?
- Do you base who your friends with by God's standards or by the worlds?
- What areas have you been letting people around you influence in a negative way you and how can you change this?

Health Check ✓

- Do you set a good example for your friends in regards to taking care of your body and mind?

Takeaways

- Follow those who follow Christ; they will less likely lead you into compromising situations
- God has called you to be defined by the amazing person He created. Don't let the world define you by what you own
- Make sure the people you are around value more than what they can accumulate here
- Choose your friends wisely and inspire those who you come in contact with every day
- Seek God on whom to spend your time with
- Ask God to guide your choices and to bring like-minded individuals into your life

Possessions Day 6

Your Time Is Your Treasure

We are on the last day of our possessions topic! I hope you have been enjoying learning about yourself as we've traveled through the word of God. Tomorrow's devotion will be a self-reflection on all six devotions and a time for you to think back on which one has made the most significant impact on you so far. Here's where will be reading from today:

Reading — Matthew 25:1-13 (NIV)

At that time the kingdom of heaven will be like ten virgins who took their lamps and went out to meet the bridegroom. Five of them were foolish, and five were wise. The foolish ones took their lamps but did not take any oil with them. The wise ones, however, took oil in jars along with their lamps. The bridegroom was a long time in coming, and they all became drowsy and fell asleep.

At midnight the cry rang out: 'Here's the bridegroom! Come out to meet him!'

Then all the virgins woke up and trimmed their lamps. The foolish ones said to the wise, 'Give us some of your oil; our lamps are going out.'

'No,' they replied, 'there may not be enough for both us and you. Instead, go to those who sell oil and buy some for yourselves.'

But while they were on their way to buy the oil, the bridegroom arrived. The virgins who were ready went in with him to the wedding banquet. And the door was shut.

Later the others also came. 'Lord, Lord,' they said, 'open the door for us!'

"But he replied, 'Truly I tell you, I don't know you.'

"Therefore keep watch, because you do not know the day or the hour."

Rarely do we as people and more importantly, Christians, look at time as a possession or resource. In this parable, we see ten women that had the same amount of time and ability to get the oil before the bridegroom came. Some took the necessary steps to be prepared, and some did not. Because half of the women did not view time as valuable, they put off completing the task until it was too late. We also can represent these women at times in our own lives. God has given each one of us different experiences and different responsibilities in this life. We all have different talents, abilities, and resources, but God requires the same thing from each of us; obedience. God asks us to use what we have, and the time He has given us, to live a life that bears fruit; meaning that we do something worth wild with all that we have. Since God is the one who created us and therefore gave us our unique abilities, it would be in our best interest to go to Him and seek after what He has designed us to do with our talents. When we seek after what He has destined us to do, we save ourselves resources that we might have wasted. This can only be done when we start viewing each and every second of every day as invaluable and as an opportunity to do the most with the life that has been given to us. It is also important to remember that timing is everything. We can miss out on opportunities and blessings that God may have for us because the steps that needed to be taken before the breakthrough were uncomfortable, inconvenient, or time-consuming. It is easy for us to squander our blessings, always asking for more from God when really what He wants is for us to use what He has already provided. How can we be trusted with more if we don't handle the little we already have with care? Time is one of our most precious possessions. It reveals who we are and eventually what we will have.

Self Reflection

- What are three things God has been calling you to do?
- What are some of the gifts and talents God has given you? Are you using them correctly?
- Have you asked God what He would have you do with what He has already blessed you with?

Health Check ✓

- God tells us that our body is a temple and we are to treasure and take care of it. Do you misuse or abuse the body and mind God has given you regarding:- food - music/ movies - books/magazines

Takeaways

- Don't ask God for more, ask Him to show you how to utilize what He has already blessed you with
- Doing nothing is just as bad as doing the wrong thing. Utilize the time God has given you

- to the fullest by asking seeking His plans for your life
- God created you with a specific life plan, ask Him to guide your steps so you can start living the life you were destined to

Possessions Day 7

Weekly Reflection

We've come to a close on our first week of devotions, and it is time to reflect. Take this time to think and answer the questions below and make sure to pray and ask God to reveal himself to you and what He wants you to take away from this topic as well. I hope you've enjoyed your first week and I cannot wait until tomorrow to continue this journey with you!

Reflection :

1. What passage in the Bible and devotion spoke to you the most? What stood out for you?
2. What can you take away from this week's topic of possessions and apply to your life starting now?
3. What has God been speaking to you as you read through each passage this week?
4. Before you pray, write out some of your prayer concerns that you need God to help you with in regards to helping shape the person you want to become
5. Have you given your life to Christ? Is this something that you believe you should do?

Prayer Concerns :

Beauty Intro

Last week all of our devotions surrounded how we defined ourselves with what we own, this week we are going to reflect on how we define ourselves by how we look. I'm sure we as women are all aware that beauty standards over the years have just gotten bigger, crazier, and more unrealistic. There is a product, cream, and procedure created for every part of our body. Companies will tell us that we are perfect the way that we are, and in the same breath sell us a product that will somehow make us "better." I have struggled and still do struggle with recognizing my own beauty and not being afraid to embrace and love myself. We see everything wrong and nothing right. We see the things we don't like as "imperfections" rather than how we were created. There is nothing wrong with improvement, but it seems our efforts have leaned more towards the physical aspect of self-improvement and less of a focus on our character traits and habits; which need to be taken into consideration when looking to improve in any way. These untouched areas that will be addressed throughout this week shine a light on what is needed to grow into the women of God we were meant to be. I know that we've all heard the speech about inward and outward beauty, but the problem nowadays is not necessarily about wanting to look or feel beautiful, but rather WHAT we consider beautiful and what we are willing to do, say, or act like, to fulfill that set standard. This week's devotions will be focusing on what God defines a beautiful woman as. It's time to look past the fixed standard and dig deeper into who we indeed can be.

"Your beauty should not come from outward adornment, such as elaborate hairstyles and the

wearing of gold jewelry or fine clothes. Rather, it should be that of your inner self, the unfading beauty of a gentle and quiet spirit, which is of great worth in God's sight."

1 Peter 3:3-4 (NIV)

Beauty Day 1

Knowledgeable Fear

Today we are going to be looking at women who fear God. Now I know sometimes when you hear the word fear you think of being frightened or afraid, and you wouldn't be wrong! However, I also want you to use the word *wise* when you think about anyone, not just women, who decide to fear God. I use the word decide because it is a choice to talk, hear, and most importantly listen, to God. Hearing and listening are two different skills. We can listen to good advice all day long, but applying it to our lives, is where wisdom comes into play. When we go to God for clarity about our lives that is us being knowledgeable enough to understand that our choices will be of much better quality when letting God direct them. He created everyone in this world and therefore knows what is best for them. However, when we not only go to God for guidance but also put daily action behind what we have been told, that is when we reach beyond just knowing what to do and show that we are wise enough to apply it to our everyday lives. When we try to live outside who God created us to be and what He has instructed us to do it is like clay telling a potter what to mold it in to. Here is an example from my own life:

I loved to go out with my friends when I was in university and college. Now there is nothing wrong with going out, but when the activities involve drinking and going to nightclubs, that conflicts with the women of God that I was and still am trying become. Every time I went out the next day I felt horrible. Everything about going out was a waste of time, and I always regretted it, but for some reason, the sin in me kept wanting to go. Saying no to certain events with them was super hard for me! I knew with my whole heart that participating in those types of activities was not helping me to grow into the person that I wanted to become, but the flesh is weak! I read in the Bible countless times where it spoke about staying away from those types of activities and the harm they bring, but for some reason through all of the knowledge that I had heard over and over again, I still kept making the same mistake. This is where the fear of God comes into play. When you genuinely have a deep, meaningful relationship with God and you truly know who he is, it becomes almost impossible to live the same way you did before. I realized that God did not want me to rid my life of certain activities because He was trying to ruin my fun. When you understand who God is and your relationship with Him is more than a Sunday morning church service, you will then be able to see why God warns you against being a part of certain activities that others would deem just good fun or even reasonable. When you chose to yield yourself to God and genuinely spend time making a relationship with Him, you will better understand yourself and the world around you. A wise woman does not follow after others but instead recognizes there is more to life and she has more to offer and then seeks after that life which calls her to be more. God only has the best for us. He created a special and unique plan for our lives, but somewhere down the line we let others define who we are as women and cheapen the beautiful creation that God has intended us to be. Be wise and fear God. Fear does not just mean being afraid, it is also understanding and respecting that God knows best and being smart enough to obey what he says. God will never force you to listen, but he did create you, form you in your mother's womb, and knows what is best for your life. He can have an incredible impact on your life if you are wise and let Him show you who He called you to be.

Let's look at some verses from the Bible about women who fear God. As you read them underline critical words that stick out to you and write down what you think of each one.

Charm is deceitful, and beauty is fleeting, but a woman who fears the LORD is to be praised.

Proverbs 31:30 (NIV)

Humility is the fear of the Lord; its wages are riches and honor and life.

Proverbs 22:4 (NIV)

The Lord delights in those who fear Him; who put their hope in His unfailing love

Psalm 147:11 (NIV)

Trust in the LORD with all your heart, and lean not on your own understanding.

Proverbs 3:5 (NIV)

The fear of the LORD is the beginning of knowledge, but fools despise wisdom and instruction

Proverbs 1:7 (NIV)

He must increase, but I must decrease.

John 3:30 (KJV)

How did you feel after reading these verses? If you are confused and want to know more about fearing God, pray! He is just waiting for you to seek him and ask questions. Seek out individuals, churches, youth groups, etc. that are around you and get involved in learning more about Christ. Even if you don't have the right words to say, go to him anyways. He will reveal Himself in a way that is unique and in a way that you can understand. I challenge you to seek God more and more in your everyday life. During my time with God in the morning, I pray that he continues to reveal Himself to me and to keep filling me with His knowledge and wisdom. I can see such a dramatic difference in who I am and how I carry myself, and you can too. I wanted the topic of having fear and respect for our Heavenly Father to be the first one of our week because it really does shape every other lesson we will be looking at. The Bible is full of God's wisdom and guidance for our lives. Everything we will touch on this coming week is about allowing ourselves to be open to the wise words that God has spoken! Like one of the verses above says: "the fear of the Lord is the beginning of knowledge." If you plan on making serious changes to your mind and body, you need to fear and respect God's Word and have an open heart to what He has to say to you.

Self Reflection:

- Do you fear and respect God enough to listen to his wisdom? Why or Why not?
- I too struggle with not just hearing but listening to God's wisdom with specific issues in my life. Like my problem with my friends, what areas do you not adhere to the advice and knowledge of God?
- Thinking about the daily activities in your life, do you know what God's Word says about them or are you living based off of how you feel and think about them?

Health Check ✓

- Do you listen to God about what you eat or what you spend your time doing?

Takeaways

- God does not ask us to give up or get rid of certain things because He wants to punish us; He created everything and everyone and knows what is best for us. It is our job to trust in His unconditional love and let it guide our everyday decisions.
- God wants to give you the very best life; one that will last an eternity! Seek Him and what he has for you.
- We make most of our mistakes just going off of what we feel, think, or what others tell us to do. Spend time seeking God and ask what He wants you to do. His will is always to benefit you.
- God wants you to grow! He wants you to become better and accomplish more than you ever thought possible!

Beauty Day 2

Go With God's Guidance

Welcome Back, I hope you are enjoying your mind and body transformation! Today we are going to be discussing how we are temples of God. A temple can also be referred to as a dwelling place or a place for worship. In the Bible, our bodies are described as "temples of the Holy Spirit." I know for the longest time I did not fully understand what that precisely meant, so for anyone like me I"ll explain. When you accept Jesus as your Lord and Saviour, God's spirit then dwells inside of you; better known as the Holy Spirit. In John 16, (NIV) Jesus speaks on His Holy Spirit saying:

"But when he, the Spirit of truth, comes, he will guide you into all the truth. He will not speak on his own; he will speak only what he hears, and he will tell you what is yet to come."

As we are all aware, Jesus had to die on the cross for us to be able to receive forgiveness and ultimately, eternal life. However Jesus did not want to leave us without guidance in our everyday lives and struggles (we see Jesus explain this later on throughout the chapter) Like I said, when we accept Jesus as our Lord and Saviour, we also receive His Holy Spirit. The Holy Spirit is here to help with our choices and decisions. He teaches and leads each of us in a personal way so that we are able to fulfill the will of God. He convicts us when we are wrong, guides when we are confused, and comforts when we are scared or lonely. How blessed are we that God did not leave us to try and decipher this world on our own! His overwhelming knowledge and wisdom are given to every believer to continually direct our actions so that we can make the best choices for our lives.

I've said all of this to help us understand our Bible reading today.

Reading — 1 Corinthians 2:6-15 (NIV)

"We do, however, speak a message of wisdom among the mature, but not the wisdom of this age or of the rulers of this age, who are coming to nothing. No, we declare God's wisdom, a mystery that has been hidden and that God destined for our glory before time began. None of the rulers of this age understood it, for if they had, they would not have crucified the Lord of glory. However, as it is written:

"What no eye has seen, what no ear has heard, and what no human mind has conceived, the things God has prepared for those who love him. These are the things God has revealed to us by his Spirit. The Spirit searches all things, even the deep things of God. For who knows a person's thoughts except their own spirit within them? In the same way, no one knows the thoughts of God except the Spirit of God. What we have received is not the spirit of the world, but the Spirit who is from God, so that we may understand what God has freely given us. This is what we speak, not in words taught us by human wisdom but in words taught by the Spirit, explaining spiritual realities with Spirit-taught words. The person without the Spirit does not accept the things that come from the Spirit of God but considers them foolishness, and cannot understand them because they are discerned only through the Spirit. The person with the Spirit makes judgments about all things, but such a person is not subject to merely human judgments.

The Holy Spirit is one of the most essential and vital blessings that God has given to His faithful followers. I use the word faithful because it is crucial to understand that to be able to hear and utilize the Holy Spirit's wisdom and guidance, we have to continually develop our relationship with God. God can only meet you as far as you decide to go. If we chose to live as the world lives; to value what they value, their lifestyle become louder than the Holy Spirits. God cannot abide and dwell in a place that is unholy, worldly, fleshly, and sinful. God speaks so adamantly on how we present and treat ourselves as He too is a part of us.

"But he that is joined unto the Lord is one spirit."

1 Corinthians 6:17 says: (KJV)

The way that we treat and present our bodies is so significant to God:

Know ye not that your bodies are the members of Christ? Shall I then take the members of Christ, and make them the members of an harlot? God forbid.

1 Corinthians 6:15 (NIV)

So what are some ways that we mistreat the body that God abides in, to be deemed "beautiful" by the world's standards?

Sex/ Sexualizing Ourselves:

I wanted to briefly touch on a predominant area that we diminish and degrade who God created us to be and the home that He lives in. God calls us to be holy, pure and righteous to name a few; He calls us to reflect Him. As women these days many of us have not presented ourselves in this manner and have either been the one to encourage a different lifestyle or are merely the ones that blindly follow those who have chosen to live outside the will of God. What many of us consider beautiful, appealing, or the right way to live these days is demonstrated in a variety of ways. Those who chose to be promiscuous (sexually active outside of marriage) are considered revolutionary. Those who desire to reveal or display their bodies are deemed confident, sexy, beautiful, and ultimately attractive. These appealing words are put in front of flawed unsuitable actions that can lead us to believe they are right and acceptable. Many then embrace these actions because they too want to feel that same sense of beauty from themselves and ultimately others. The reality is this: it is the belief (that has been forced upon us in many ways) that these actions will make us more appealing that drive us towards pursuing them. It does not mean they are right but rather an idea that has been accepted over time.

Because we are daily bombarded with these beliefs either from celebrities, ads, people around us, etc. many times we may actually begin to adhere to them. God knows we can be more, are worth more, and how much we are selling ourselves short when we give into the standards of the world. Our bodies and what we can do with them have made up so much of who we are for far too long. What most of us women forget or maybe never learned, is that true confidence and self-love does not come from stripping ourselves from everything we are or who we were made to be so that those around us can consider us beautiful, confident, sexy, or anything else of that likeness. God sees us as so much more than sexual objects; as things to have fun with for a night before moving on to a newer model. When we recognize that our worth is not in how we look, but through God's original and unique design for us, we will be able to be confident whether we are in a bikini or full Amish attire. We need to take back the definition of what beauty truly means. Let's look at how God's Word describes a beautiful woman; I think you may be a bit surprised!

I also want the women to dress modestly, with decency and propriety, adorning themselves, not with elaborate hairstyles or gold or pearls or expensive clothes

1 Timothy 2:9 (NIV)

She is clothed with strength and dignity

Proverbs 31:25 (NIV)

But the LORD said to Samuel, "Do not consider appearance or height, for I have rejected him. The LORD does not look at the things man looks at. Man looks at the outward appearance, but the LORD looks at the heart."

1 Samuel 16:7 (NIV)

For physical training is of some value, but godliness has value for all things, holding promise for both the present life and the life to come

1 Timothy 4:8 (NIV)

Your heart became proud on account of your beauty, and you corrupted your wisdom because of your splendor.

Ezekiel 28:17 (NIV)

Flee from sexual immorality. All other sins a person commits are outside the body, but whoever sins sexually, sins against their own body

1 Corinthians 6:18 (NIV)

It is God's will that you should be sanctified: that you should avoid sexual immorality; that each of you should learn to control your own body in a way that is holy and honorable, not in passionate lust like the pagans, who do not know God;

1 Thessalonians 4:3-5 (NIV)

Flee the evil desires of youth and pursue righteousness, faith, love, and peace, along with those who call on the Lord out of a pure heart.

2 Timothy 2:22 (NIV)

We will never feel content or fulfilled when we sexualize ourselves because it is not the way that God designed us to find fulfillment. It is easy to enjoy sin, but once you truly experience the life Christ has for you and understand the person He has called you to be, the difference is incredible. Most of us sell our worth to the world for next to nothing. Real fulfillment will never come from an Instagram like or a one night stand. These things do not empower you, they cheapen you. God considers you priceless, but our actions have to line up with his not the worlds for us to see who we are really meant to be.

Self Reflection

- How do you sexualize yourself?
- Do you really feel right about this or are you trying to live up to the expectations of others?

- If you do feel okay about presenting yourself this way, after reading these verses do you still feel the same way? Why or Why Not?
- What could the benefits be of adjusting your behavior to reflect the characteristics of Godly women?

Health Check ✓

- Do you prioritize the actual health of your body or are you more focused on the physical aspects? Which one do you prioritize more?

Takeaways

- The Holy Spirit wants to help guide us into women that have more to offer than our bodies; cultivate your relationship with Christ so that you can truly be fulfilled!
- Just like you would clean up your house before having people visit, clean up your heart and mind so that Christ can comfortably come in
- You are more than body parts! Strive to find worth outside of your appearance
- God sees the best version of you and has the blueprint for you to become her. Listen to the Holy Spirit so that you can be guided into all knowledge and truth.

Beauty Day 3

Your Splendor Is In Your Speech

Today we are going to be looking at our tongue! We all need to be aware of the power of our words and how they can shape the way in which people see us. As women, we have been degraded and belittled for years, so it is important not to help the cause by acting in any way that encourages the shallow empty view many have towards us. How we carry ourselves as a whole determines how and what people think of us. Now I know what many of you may be thinking; "Just because I decide to dress or talk a certain way or participate in certain activities it does not give anyone the right to assume who I am." Although that is a valid point, and the only one that truly knows who you are is Jesus, the fact remains that if you want to be known as something, then you need to look and act the part. If you saw a man wearing a police officer uniform wearing a badge and a gun, you would treat him as a police officer, and the same goes for the way in which we present ourselves. We will be treated how we are introduced. Our words can either bring life or death to our appearance. We can speak with dignity, respect, and in a wholesome manner or we can talk vulgarly and ignorantly and reap the benefits of that type of language. A wise woman understands that by speaking and dressing in a respectable manner, she is not only holding herself to a higher standard but demanding that others do as well. As women of God, we are called to be more, and we cannot do that by trying to be the same as everyone else. Let's look at some verses that touch on the tongue and the way that we should speak. As we read them, underline, star or write anything down that comes to your mind.

She speaks with wisdom, and faithful instruction is on her tongue

Proverbs 31:26 (NIV)

Whoever would love life and see good days, must keep their tongue from evil and their lips from deceitful speech

1 Peter 3:10 (NIV)

The tongue has the power of life and death

Proverbs 18:21 (NIV)

In the same way, women are to be worthy of respect, not malicious talkers but temperate and trustworthy in everything

1 Timothy 3:11 (NIV)

The words of the reckless pierce like swords, but the tongue of the wise brings healing

Proverbs 12:18 (NIV)

God requires so much from us because we were made to reflect him! He knows who we can be and what we are capable of. He also knows when we present ourselves in a way that does not honor the individuals we were made to be, our value and worth become cheapened. As women of God, we need to be striving towards having the utmost respect for ourselves in every area of our lives, from the way that we dress to the words that come out of our mouths!

Self Reflection:

- What areas of your life do you feel you have disrespected yourself?
- What areas of your life do you feel others have disrespected you?
- Do you think how you have been presenting yourself has anything to do with it?
- Are you careful with your words or do you say whatever you feel and think?
- How has what you said or how you speak shaped you negatively?
- How can you start making better choices with your words?
- Do you think the people that you surround yourself with have anything to do with how you speak?

Health Check ✓

- As we read in one of our Bible verses above, there is life and death in our tongue. Negative words and feelings not only affect you spiritually but mentally and physically as well! We need to make sure we are imparting life into ourselves with our food, words, and lifestyle so that we can live happy, healthy, peaceful lives.

Takeaways

- You cannot always control the way others view or treat you, but do your part and leave the rest to God
- If you want respect, require it! We cannot expect to be treated a certain way if we treat ourselves the exact opposite
- Our words are powerful, make sure you use them to build up others not destroy them

Beauty Day 4

Social Standards Are Not Always Suitable

Welcome Back! I know we are talking about some touchy topics, but I hope you are able to take something out of each devotion to better yourself as a woman of God. Today we are going to be discussing how we as women view men. Now I don't know about you, but almost every girl power song or message that I've heard surrounds how much we don't need to rely on men. There are also the songs that talk about the requirements men need to have or who they need to be to be deemed worthy to be in our lives. Although I agree to some extent with these statements, I have also noticed a pattern that we have started to view men as disposable. Now before you completely disagree with me, hear me out! The opinions and beliefs of this day and age have helped create a very confident but cold type of women. We put so much pressure on ourselves to look and act a certain way and also put that same pressure on the men in our lives to fulfill our impossible standards. Like I mentioned previously, we are told exactly how we should act towards men, what we deserve, what they should bring to our lives, how they should look, and if they don't meet the criteria, that we can do better and we deserve better. Although there is absolutely nothing wrong with having standards, we also need to remember the way in which Christ calls us to view our relationships.

Reading — 1 Corinthians 13:4-13 (NIV)

Love is patient, love is kind. It does not envy, it does not boast, it is not proud.5 It does not dishonor others, it is not self-seeking, it is not easily angered, it keeps no record of wrongs. 6 Love does not delight in evil but rejoices with the truth. 7 It always protects, always trusts, always hopes, always perseveres. Love never fails. But where there are prophecies, they will cease; where there are tongues, they will be stilled; where there is knowledge, it will pass away. For we know in part and we prophesy in part, but when completeness comes, what is in part disappears. When I was a child, I talked like a child, I thought like a child, I reasoned like a child. When I became a man, I put the ways of childhood behind me. For now, we see only a reflection as in a mirror; then we shall see face to face. Now I know in part; then I shall know fully, even as I am fully known. And now these three remain faith, hope, and love. But the greatest of these is love.

During His time here on earth, Jesus spoke about what the greatest and most important commandment is, and that is to love others. We are told to love through everything and the way in which Christ loves us; unconditionally. The problem with most relationships today is that they are based on conditions. If the person we are with does not look or appear the way in which we want him to, we are quick to write off the relationship instead of remembering the greatest commandment. When we learn that our value and others are not based on what this world tells us is necessary, we will be able to let go of what holds us back from having the lasting and meaningful relationships that we all desire. Our story books, movies, magazines, music, and sometimes even our roles models as women, have told us to find our value and worth in our beauty and what we have, and in turn require these same conditions from the person that we are with. We go into relationships with preconceived standards and biases, and none involve the qualities presented in 1 Corinthians: Patient, kind, does not boast, is not proud, is not self-seeking, not easily angered, keeps no record of wrongdoings; these are all the things Jesus describes as showing love. Jesus goes on to say that love ALWAYS protects, preserves, hopes, and trusts. Jesus does not mean to love based on your past experiences or others past experiences either. We are told to love ALWAYS and with no limit. When we take a loving spirit into our relationships rather than basing it off of fleeting physical attributes, we learn what a relationship is indeed. A relationship is two people deciding every day to love the other person no matter what they have or do not have. When both individuals are willing to withstand the easy and challenging situations, it takes off a lot of pressure to live up to impossible physical and materialistic standards that we have been told must be present in the relationship to be deemed acceptable.

Self Reflection

- What impossible standards do place on your partner?
- Are these materialistic or physical?
- Do you think they reflect the way in which God calls us to love?
- Do you focus more on what you are getting from your relationship or what you are giving?
- Do you think this type of mindset is helping or hindering your relationship?

Health Check ✓

- Having healthy relationships is part of living a happy life. Do you openly and honestly communicate with your husband/boyfriend about things that are bothering or upsetting you? Don't forget to take your concerns to the Lord in prayer first so that He can show you a solution as well.

Takeaways:

- God looks at our heart not what we see on the outside, spend more time loving who you are with, not what they could be or what they can give to you
- Don't look at what you don't have, look at the person you are with and what they bring to your life
- Focus more on what you can give in your relationship rather than what you are getting

Beauty Day 5

Pretty Purposeful

We are almost finished our second week of devotions! I hope you are learning as much as me and are enjoying this topic. Now that we have discussed all of the different ways that we are beautiful inside and out, I want to talk about the way in which we use our beauty. God has given us as women such a unique and irreplaceable role in the lives of those around us. He has made us with abilities and character traits that are unlike anyone else. We are loving, nurturing, compassionate, forgiving, individuals to name a few! These inherent traits that we as women possess are some of the best ways that we show our beauty in our daily lives, however, there are ways that we misuse and devalue our inner and outer beauty. For this topic, I am going to split up the devotion into two days and talk about three women who had different situations but the same opportunity to use the immense amount of beauty that God had given them to better the lives of those around them. One chose to do so, and the others decided to use their vision to damage and destroy themselves and others. The women that we will be discussing today is Esther. Now maybe some of you reading have never heard the story of Esther so I will give a recap of her life and the blessing she was to the people around her. Esther was a young Jewish girl, and at this time the Jewish people had been driven out of their home, Israel and were forced to flee to Persia. She lived with her cousin Mordechai who was also a leader of the Jews in Persia at this time. Esther was chosen by the king to become his new queen but had never shared her Jewish background with anyone as Mordecai had told her to conceal it because of the hate some had towards Jewish people. Let's start our reading and learn all about this amazing woman of God and how she saved so many lives by using what God had given her properly.

Reading — Esther 2: 7-17 (NIV)

Mordecai had a cousin named Hadassah, whom he had brought up because she had neither father nor mother. This young woman, who was also known as Esther, had a lovely figure and was beautiful. Mordecai had taken her as his own daughter when her father and mother died.

When the king's order and edict had been proclaimed, (to take a new wife) many young women were brought to the citadel of Susa and put under the care of Hegai. Esther also was taken to the king's palace and entrusted to Hegai, who had charge of the harem. She pleased him and won his favor. Immediately he provided her with her beauty treatments and exceptional food. He assigned to her seven female attendants selected from the king's palace and moved her and her attendants into the best place in the harem.

Esther had not revealed her nationality and family background, because Mordecai had forbidden her to do so. Every day he walked back and forth near the courtyard of the harem to find out how Esther was and what was happening to her.

Before a young woman's turn came to go into King Xerxes, she had to complete twelve months of beauty treatments prescribed for the women, six months with oil of myrrh and six with perfumes and cosmetics. She would not return to the king unless he was pleased with her and summoned her by name.

Now the king was attracted to Esther more than to any of the other women, and she won his favor and approval more than any of the other virgins. So he set a royal crown on her head and made her queen instead of Vashti. And the king gave a great banquet, Esther's banquet, for all his nobles and officials. He proclaimed a holiday throughout the provinces and distributed gifts with royal liberality.

** Esther did not know it at this time, but God was showing her an immense amount of favor so that she would be able to save her people in the months to come.

Reading — Esther 3:1-5 (NIV)

"After these events, King Xerxes honored Haman [one of his servants] elevating him and giving him a seat of honor higher than that of all the other nobles. All the royal officials at the king's gate knelt down and paid homage to Haman, for the king had commanded this concerning him. But Mordecai would not kneel down or pay him honor.

Then the royal officials at the king's gate asked Mordecai, "Why do you disobey the king's command?" Day after day they spoke to him, but he refused to comply. Therefore they told Haman about it to see whether Mordecai's behavior would be tolerated, for he had said them he was a Jew.

When Haman saw that Mordecai would not kneel down or pay him honor, he was enraged. Yet having learned who Mordecai's people were, he scorned the idea of killing only Mordecai. Instead, Haman looked for a way to destroy all Mordecai's people, the Jews, throughout the whole kingdom of Xerxes."

Because of Haman's hate towards Mordecai, he convinced the king to kill every Jew in Persia. Mordecai told Esther about this decree that would be followed out shortly and said to her that she needed to go to the King and ask him to spare the lives of her people. Esther was terrified to do this as no one was allowed to go before the king unless they were called by him and the penalty to this crime was death. The beauty and charm that God had given Esther helped her become the Queen of Persia, but now she had the choice to utilize these gifts for more than just herself. Esther decided to go to in front of the king anyways and took the risk of being killed. The king spared Esther, and when she finally told him all Haman's plan to kill her people, he had him murdered and canceled the decree against the Jews. As I said before, God blessed Esther with not only beauty, but charm, strength, and courage. She decided to use her talents and gifts not only to benefit her own life but to save and benefit the lives of others. We as women have the same opportunity to do what Esther did. We can use what God has given us to build up and better our lives and the lives of those around us, or we can demean, diminish and destroy ourselves by using what we have in the wrong way.

Self Reflection

- What ways do you use your beauty?
- Do you think these ways are pleasing to the Lord?
- Are these vain pursuits?
- How can you use what God has given you to benefit others?
- Like Esther, God has given each of us something to do with your gifts/talents? Have you asked Him what that is for you?
- If you already know, have you began to live it in your daily life?

Health Check ✓

- When we focus too much on our outside beauty, it is easy
  to forget about the way we look and feel on the inside. Are
  you nurturing and caring for who you are as much as you
  nurture and care about what you look like?

Takeaways

- Our soul is the only part of us that does not grow old, fade,
  or lose its beauty, make choices that benefit and ultimately
  decide where you will live eternally
- God has given you your appearance to bring glory to him!
- Don't cheapen the beautiful creation God has made you be
  by living up to the norms of this world.

Beauty Day 6

Pretty Purposeful Devotion

This is the continuation of yesterday's topic regarding the way in which we use our beauty! I think this topic is one of the most important ones that we will talk about throughout this entire month. As we go into this next devotion, let's remember the importance of the way in which we use what God has given us. Let's continue to grow into beautiful, strong women of God and talk about two women who used their beauty in very wrong ways.

Jezebel:

In the Bible, there is a woman by the name of Jezebel mentioned, and from what we know about her she was not a very Godly woman. Jezebel was a princess and eventually became the Queen of Israel; however she did not build up her husband in God; in fact, she did the exact opposite. Jezebel used her beauty and cunning words to convince her husband to forsake God and serve false gods such as Baal. This lead to numerous problems throughout the land of Israel including death and famine. Like I said previously, women were created specially by God with a specific set of abilities and character traits. Jezebel decided to use hers to encourage rebellion and disobedience towards God. Let's look at some verses that talk about just how detrimental this woman was.

"Nevertheless, I have this against you: You tolerate that woman Jezebel, who calls herself a prophet. By her teaching, she misleads my servants into sexual immorality and the eating of food sacrificed to idols."

Revelations 2:20 (NIV)

And when Jehu came to Jezreel, Jezebel heard of it; and she painted her face, and tired her head, and looked out at a window

2 Kings 9:30 (KJV)

I wanted us to look at these two verses in particular because the first displays the anger of God towards those that chose to use their beauty to not only dishonor him with their actions but also influence others to participate in activities that are against His Holy Word.

The second verse is taken from 2 Kings, and it is at the time where Jezebel's reign in Israel was coming to a close, and a man named Jehu was coming to kill her. When she saw that he was coming, Jezebel again tried to save herself with her beauty and dressed in makeup and beautiful clothing to try and persuade Jehu not to kill her. This, however, did not work, and she was finally removed as the queen of Israel. Even when guilty, Jezebel tried to use her charm and beauty to help her but eventually, that was not enough, and the same goes for us today. Jezebel was put into a position of power and could have used this to become a great woman of God, but instead, she decided to use what was given to her physically and materialistically to destroy her life and countless other lives as well.

Delilah:

The last women we are going to look at today is Delilah. This woman was a philistine, and because of her beauty, a mighty man of God married her. This is significant because the Philistines were against God's people and were always trying to destroy them. Samson knew that but only focused on Delilah's beauty not on who she was as a person. God gave Samuel the gift of strength; no man or beast could harm or kill Samson because God's favor was upon Him. God told Samson that his power would remain with him as long as he did not cut his hair. Samson's parents warned him against marrying Delilah, but because of her beauty, he did not listen. Let's read our passages today.

Reading — Judges 14:1-4 (NIV)

Samson went down to Timnah and saw there a young Philistine woman. **2** When he returned, he said to his father and mother, "I have seen a Philistine woman in Timnah; now get her for me as my wife."

His father and mother replied, "Isn't there an acceptable woman among your relatives or among all our people? Must you go to the uncircumcised Philistines to get a wife?"

But Samson said to his father, "Get her for me. She's the right one for me." (His parents did not know that this was from the Lord, who was seeking an occasion to confront the Philistines; for at that time they were ruling over Israel.)

Judges 15:4- 21 (NIV)

Sometime later, he fell in love with a woman in the Valley of Sorek whose name was Delilah. The rulers of the Philistines went to her and said, "See if you can lure him into showing you the secret of his great strength and how we can overpower him so we may tie him up and subdue him. Each one of us will give you eleven hundred shekels of silver."

So Delilah said to Samson, "Tell me the secret of your great strength and how you can be tied up and subdued."

Then she said to him, "How can you say, 'I love you,' when you won't confide in me? This is the third time you have made a fool of me and haven't told me the secret of your great strength." With such nagging, she prodded him day after day until he was sick to death of it.

So he told her everything. "No razor has ever been used on my head," he said, "because I have been a Nazirite dedicated to God from my mother's womb. If my head were shaved, my strength would leave me, and I would become as weak as any other man."

When Delilah saw that he had told her everything, she sent word to the rulers of the Philistines, "Come back once more; he has told me everything." So the rulers of the Philistines returned with the silver in their hands. After putting him to sleep on her lap, she called for someone to shave off the seven braids of his hair, and so began to subdue him. And his strength left him.

Then she called, "Samson, the Philistines are upon you!"

He awoke from his sleep and thought, "I'll go out as before and shake myself free." But he did not know that the Lord had left him.

Then the Philistines seized him, gouged out his eyes and took him down to Gaza. Binding him with bronze shackles, they set him to grinding grain in the prison."

As we can see from these passages, Samson decided to marry Delilah with very little knowledge of who she was and without approval from God. He allowed Delilah to persuade him into revealing his secret to his strength which ended up leading to his destruction. Although he lost his power and was captured, God gave Samson back his strength one more time to kill many of the Philistines and their temple. When we judge people based solely off of how they physically look we can make detrimental mistakes in our lives. A mindset focused more on physical beauty leaves little room to nurture Godly character in our daily lives.

This world can push ideas on us of what we need to do to feel "good" about ourselves. They tell us that wearing revealing clothes, masks of makeup, and being open to giving multiple people the most private parts of ourselves will make us feel our best. Many of us will say that we genuinely enjoy these aspects of life, but if this was indeed the way in which we were meant to find our fulfillment God would not require more from us. These shallow habits that cause temporary joy due to the worldly reaction we obtain from them leave us feeling that if we do not have, look, dress, or act this way we are somehow not as worthy as those who do. God has so much more for each of us, and when we decide to use our beauty and talents to dishonor ourselves or others, we devalue the precious person we are.

Self Reflection:

- Are you like Delilah and Jezebel? Do you use your beauty to manipulate those around you?
- Do you rely on your beauty to feel confident or to get what you want? Why?
- Is your worth found in the way that you look, or who God created you to be?

Health Check ✓

- Do you bring others along with you to live healthier happier lives?

Takeaways:

- We are more than what the world says we are! Ask God to show you how much more you have to offer to yourself and others
- Don't use how you look to mistreat or manipulate others
- As the word of God says beauty is fleeting, and charm is deceptive, concentrate on the things in life that matter, not on the opinions that others have of you physically

Beauty Day 7

Weekly Reflection

Our second week of strengthening our mind and body has ended. I love learning more about the areas that we as women struggle with and practical ways we can better ourselves in our daily lives. As we move into the next topic, take some time to really reflect on what we have learned and where you can continue to grow and make changes. I love learning with you, and I cannot wait to share next week's topic with you! Blessings,
-Yvonne

Weekly Reflection :

1. What passage and devotion spoke to you the most? Why?
2. What can you take away from this week's topic of possessions and apply to your life starting now?
3. What has God been speaking to you as you read through each passage this week?
4. Before you pray, write out some of your prayer concerns that you need God to help you with in regards to helping shape the person you want to become

Prayer Concerns :

Self Esteem Intro

I heard a quote once that said, "Imagine if women woke up tomorrow and decided to love their bodies, how many companies would go out of business?"

Now to me this relates far past companies and far past our bodies, and involves many other areas of women's lives. To me, it is not just our physical bodies that we detest, it is a vast majority of other areas that we find something to dislike. Our dislikes, from our hair to our laugh and everything in between, comes from a place inside of us. It comes from a place of not being able to accept who we are because we are told and tell ourselves that there is always something that needs to be changed and something not to like. The reason why I wanted to take a whole week of our one month journey together and discuss self-esteem is that our lack of it seems to shape our everyday lives. When we don't like the way we SEE ourselves, how we feel about ourselves begins to change. We become more susceptible to what others think or say about us because we most likely already believe, and perhaps repeat, similar negative statements to ourselves. New negative comments that arise either from others or ourselves could also be accepted as accurate due to already having a low outlook on who we are. When we begin to feel and think of ourselves in this way, we begin to allow the people around us or those that we deem "worthy" enough, to change what we should focus on.

Women especially are told that they are not good enough, and the more that we believe that from the media, society, and many times, even the relationships that we have, the more self-harm we inflict. When we have not spent time developing ourselves with God, it is easy for people to come along and dictate who we should be and how we should act. Our self-esteem issues push us toward wanting acceptance from others. We allow so many people to tell us what should be of importance to us, that we forget about what we want and most importantly who God originally created us to be. We are not meant to fit into the same cookie cutter box as the next women. We are all beautifully unique. The Bible says:

"I am fearfully and wonderfully made." (NIV)

I have learned and continue to learn throughout my life that God has made a specific plan and purpose for each and every one of us. No two are alike, but each one is perfect for who we are and who He created us to be. When we start trying to become a copy of someone else we miss out on everything He designed each of us individually to do on this earth. You will never fully accomplish the destiny God created explicitly for you trying to fulfill someone's else's. Our Heavenly Father can transform you into the best version of yourself through a relationship with Him. His direction is never wrong, and it never leads you down a path that was not meant for you. As we explore more about self-esteem this week, ask God to open your heart and your mind to what you have been allowing others to dictate in your life.

Self Esteem Day 1

God's Great View of You

Welcome back! We are at the beginning of a new week and a new topic! I hope you are enjoying each devotion and can continue to apply it your life as we go.

It's easy to forget just how special we are. Life seems to magnify all that is wrong with us, what we perhaps don't have, what hasn't been accomplished yet, and so much more. Sometimes we can begin to think through broken promises, failed relationships, or the hurtful actions of others, that there is something wrong with us. Sometimes perhaps we are the problem, but there are many situations that we inherently blame ourselves for when in actuality had nothing to do with how someone else decided to treat us. None of us are perfect and at many times in our lives can purposely or unintentionally hurt others. The only one who will never hurt or betray us is God. He is never out to get us, trying to be mean, trying to withhold good, or acting out of the selfish, self-centered behavior. His intentions always have been and remain perfect for you and me. Many times we can begin to feel sorry about who we are because we have allowed other people to define how we should think about ourselves; forgetting to look to the very one that created us. There have been times in my own life where God has picked me up from dark places, anxious thoughts, and feelings, and renewed my spirit in His love for me. He reminds me of my worth, value, and all I am in him. In Christ and Christ alone am I secure and happy; I am whole. Everyone, even yourself sees only parts of you. It can be hard to see the good when sometimes we can't even find it. I found myself when I found Christ. He revealed who I am and who I was meant to be. God sees each of us in the most beautiful way, not the harsh critics that we judge ourselves against. He doesn't have unrealistic beauty standards or expectations, but instead, he wants to show us how beautiful we were created to be. Today I want you to understand what your Heavenly Father thinks about you and how He sees you. Here are some eternal truths about how special you are to God.

You Are One Of A Kind:

For you created my inmost being: you knit me together in my mother's body.

I praise you because I am fearfully and wonderfully made;

Your works are wonderful. I know that full well

My frame was not hidden from you when I was made in the secret place, when I was woven together in the depths of the earth.

Psalm 139: 13-15 (NIV)

God did not make you like anyone else. He made you unique in every single way possible. Just like there are no two snowflakes alike, there is no other person in this world like you! God wants to use who He made you to be to accomplish amazing things. You can't fulfill your life's purpose if you aren't true to yourself

You Are Not An Accident:

Your eyes saw my unformed body; all the days ordained for me were written in your book before one of them came to be.

Psalm 139: 16 (NIV)

Your hands made me and formed me; give me understanding to learn your commands

Psalm 119:73 (NIV)

Before I formed you in the womb I knew you, before you were born I set you apart; I appointed you as a prophet to the nations."

Jeremiah 1:4-5 (NIV)

God did not make a mistake when He created you. He knew exactly what He was doing when he formed you and breathed the breath of life into your body. Even if your parents weren't planning on having you, God was. He created you with purpose and intent and wanted you on this Earth and eternally with Him.

You Have A Specific Purpose:

"For I know the plans I have for you" declares the Lord, "plans to prosper you and not to harm you, plans to give you a hope and a future."

Jeremiah 29:11 (NIV)

Each of you should use whatever gift you have received to serve others, as faithful stewards of God's grace in its various forms

1 Peter 4:10 (NIV)

Just like God created you perfectly unique, He created your life plan specifically to who He made you be. There are certain things only YOU can fulfill because you have the right character and skills to do so. Looking at what others are accomplishing does not benefit you and serves only as a distraction to what you are to be fulfilling. Daily ask God what your purpose on this earth is. He will lead you into fulfillment on this side of life and into eternity with Him!

You Are Extremely Valuable And Important To God:

How precious to me are your thoughts, God! How vast is the sum of them? Were I to count them, they would outnumber the grains of sand - when I awake, I am still with you

Psalm 139: 17-18 (NIV)

Are not two sparrows sold for a penny? Yet not one of them will fall to the ground outside your Father's care. And even the very hairs of your head are all numbered. So don't be afraid; you are worth more than many sparrows.

Matthew 10:29-31 (NIV)

He did not spare his own Son but gave him for us all

Romans 8:32 (NIV)

The most amazing gift that we have ever been given is eternal life through the sacrifice Jesus made on the cross. He died so that we could be free from our sins and therefore justified to live eternally in paradise. Pastor Rick Warren wrote in his book "A Purpose Driven Life." "God could not imagine eternity without you." That is how special you are to God. It pleased Him to send His Son to die for us because we now have the priceless gift of living with Him forever. God doesn't need anything from us, He created us because it pleased Him, blesses us because He loves us, and sacrificed His Son because He wants us with Him forever. Whenever you feel like your life doesn't matter, remember the priceless gift God gave just for you. He was willing to send His own Son to die for your sin because He wants to spend eternity with you in paradise.

You Can Never Be More Loved And Accepted Than You Are Right Now

But God demonstrates his own love for us in this: While we were still sinners, Christ died for us

Romans 5:8 (NIV)

But you are a forgiving God, gracious and compassionate, slow to anger and abounding in love

Nehemiah 9:17 (NIV)

"And walk in the way of love, just as Christ loved us and gave himself up for us as a fragrant offering and sacrifice to God."

Ephesians 5:2 (NIV)

Sometimes we feel as if we have to earn other people's love. We think that people will not love or appreciate us if we do not look a certain way, have a specific title or career, have the right upbringing, or obtain wealth. All of these aspects are shallow and worthless to God. He does define your worth by the same standards of the world. He knows exactly how special you are because He made you! There will never be anything more you can do or possess that will change the way God feels about you. He loves you despite your sin, failures, faults, appearance, or what you have in your bank account. His love is not dependant on materialistic items or people. There is nothing you can do to earn eternal life or God's love for you, and there never has been. It never changes, and his mercy is new every day. Others may forget, hold grudges, or keep score, but when we ask Christ for forgiveness, it's as if we never sinned. Let your worth rest in the only one who sees the very best in you and is not reliant on who you are or what you have to love and treasure you! When we find our worth and value in others instead of God, we quickly forget how special we are. When others fail to recognize how amazing we are, we think this means that we are not. God does not need others to see how irreplaceably unique you are to know for Himself. He made you, loves you, and sent His Son to die for you so He could have you in His life forever!

Self Reflection

- Where have you placed your worth? (People, titles, careers, accomplishments, etc.)
- Do you feel fulfilled in the places you've put it? Why or Why Not?
- In what ways do you fail to recognize your own worth?
- Do you think others treat you the way you see yourself? How?

Health Check ✓

- Do you create your health goals based on what others value or are they more dependant on what is best for you?

Takeaways

- Get closer to your Heavenly Father! He wants to reveal the beautiful women He created you to be

- When you know God, you are able to see yourself in the most perfect light
- God doesn't look at all the things you don't have, but rather all He gave you and made you to be
- Ask God to reveal himself to you more so you can get closer to living the one who knows you best

Esteem Day 2

Disappointments & Accomplishments

Welcome back! Today we are going to be discussing our self-esteem regarding our accomplishments. We all have dreams, hopes, passions, pursuits, etc. These are usually founded when we are quite young, how we grow up, and what our parents and families want for us or have exposed us to. I know for myself growing up I always wanted to go to University and become a teacher. This was deeply rooted in my social circle. All my friends basically knew exactly what they wanted to do and how to pursue it. They held their academic future quite crucial on their list of pursuits, and they influenced me to do the same. I went to university without much of a plan and more of an interest which was to my downfall. This ended up costing me a lot of time and money. I dropped out of school early because I did not feel like I was really working towards anything other than a piece of paper that allowed me to work in a field that I wasn't even sure I wanted to. Some people understood and accepted my choice and others did not. Some encouraged me to pursue a different career and others made me feel that I had made a terrible mistake. Their opinions came from rigid viewpoints of how success is found and obtained. I remember starting to feel really bad about myself. I began to view myself and my life as embarrassing and worthless.

God has done an enormous amount work in my life and in me in regards to this. Here is what He revealed to me in these moments of self-doubt:

What this world considers an accomplishment is vastly different than what God does

If there is anything that you take out of this whole book it is this point right here:

Many of the things that we consider achievements in this life are the ideas of others.

Money, fame, education, careers, materialistic possessions, a significant other, are just some of the things that we are told portray a successful individual. God does not focus on these things to define our success. It is much more about the specific purpose He has given each of us to fulfill on this earth that is the true definition of a successful person. Because of this, success cannot be wrapped up in a few titles but rather on specific obedience to God and His Word. To many people, our lives may not scream achievement, but if we are following what God has told us to do, then we are right on track.

When Jesus came to this earth, it was not to find his worthiness in others. He understood who He was and His mission. There were times where people respected Jesus and called Him Messiah, but that was not always the case. As we know by the end of Jesus's life, they crucified and ridiculed Him. The inability for people to see who Jesus indeed was did not change that He was the Son of God and it did not break His desire to fulfill the purpose God gave to

Him. Jesus's mission was to enlighten and save the lost, then and for all eternity:

Jesus went throughout Galilee, teaching in their synagogues, proclaiming the good news of the kingdom, and healing every disease and sickness among the people.

Matthew 4:23 (NIV)

Others inability to see your worth does not change your worth, in fact, it does more harm to them than you! People will judge you prematurely or with how much respect they think you deserve, perhaps never getting to know the beautiful person you are. The Bible tells us that Jesus himself was not able to perform many miracles in the place that He was born because the people viewed Him in a low manner. They did not believe He could be the Messiah because they had grown up with Him and knew Him from when He was a boy.

Jesus said to them, 'A prophet is not without honor except in his own town, among his relatives and in his own home.' He could not do any miracles there, except lay his hands on a few sick people and heal them. He was amazed at their lack of faith."

Mark 6:4-5 (NIV)

Jesus could not save, heal, deliver, or cure countless individuals in Nazareth because they were stuck in their own viewpoint of who they thought He was and this sometimes can reflect how we treat others or how others treat us.

Many times people will view us the same way they saw Jesus, but that does not mean that we are any less of the amazing women that God has made us be and it certainly does not mean that we should live below it. We do not need to feel insecure or unhappy because others cannot see us for who we are. We are to live boldly and as new creations in Christ no matter what others think or how they may feel. It is sometimes those closest to us that hurt us the most. It is sometimes those closest to us that do not believe we could be anything more than our past mistakes. Do not let anyone rob you of the life that you can have through Christ Jesus. Go to your Heavenly Father and find your worth and value in who He made you to be.

Self Reflection

- Have you been allowing someone in your life to dictate how you see yourself or what you think you can accomplish?
- Who and Why?
- In what ways have you been holding yourself back? (past mistakes/regrets)
- What is one action that you can start doing today towards your goals?
- Have you talked to God about what His plan for your life is? If not, why?

Health Check ✓

- Are your lifestyle habits and how you treat your body dependent on how others live or how you want to live?

Takeaways

- Do not allow others to dictate what you can accomplish
- People will not always see you the way that you want them to, but that does not change who you are
- God sees the very best version of you, let his Holy Spirit transform you into that person

- God loves you and has amazing plans for your life, ask Him to reveal them to you so you can live fulfilled and content in Him!
- Never let the inability of others to see your worth. Define how you look at yourself through Christ

Relationships Day 3

Drop Your Mindset And Grab Christ's Character

The next three devotions we will be switching topics and addressing our relationships. Today, in particular, we will be discussing our relationships with men. There is so much that can be said about our relations with the opposite sex, it really could be a full week or even an entire month of devotions! The first point that I would like to address is that God loves relationships. One of the main reasons we are here on this earth is to have contact with others and especially amongst fellow believers. God created man and woman for many reasons, one of them being for the intimate relationship.

"That is why a man leaves his father and mother and is united to his wife, and they become one flesh."

Genesis 2:24 (NIV)

We are made to help, encourage, strengthen, and add joy to each other's lives. God loves and created relationship because He knows we are better together. God designed relationship and therefore tells us exactly how to have success in them. God said that the greatest commandment of all the ones He has given us is love! God is love, and therefore we too must love people and especially those who we are in a relationship with passionately and even when it is hard. Although we are instructed to love and sacrifice for others, God wants us to love and sacrifice for Him first and daily. Many times, however, we get it backwards, and we begin to love others first; inevitably showing our lack of love for Christ. We demonstrate this mainly through where we spend our time. If spending time with God, incorporating Him into every part of your day, and being obedient to Him, are not daily actions in your life, then you are just not ready for an intimate relationship. It is our biggest downfall when we decide to pursue a man without having our foundation first rooted in Christ. Why is a deep connection with Christ absolutely vital BEFORE entering into any other relationship? We will spend the remainder of the devotion discussing one of the reasons that this is so important and the next devotion discussing the last two ideas. You will complete the self-reflection, health check questions tomorrow at the end of tomorrow's reading.

1. Relationship With Christs Reveals Who You Are

Having a relationship with God allows Him to show us who we truly are. We carry so many problems into our relationships because we never fix the root of the issue; ourselves. Your self-esteem whether good or bad can become an issue in your relationship if you do not allow God to daily mold who you should be. If you view yourself as perfect or close to it, you will find it hard to believe that problems in your relationship could be your fault. You may find it hard to accept that you have character faults because of the very high view you have of yourself. I am in no way implying that women should not be confident, but I do believe that sometimes an overconfident "im perfect" attitude can cause more harm than good in our relationships. Let's look at some verses about the dangers of pride:

"In his pride, the wicked man does not seek him; in all his thoughts there is no room for God."

Psalms 10:4 (NIV)

"If anyone thinks they are something when they are not, they deceive themselves"

Galatians 6:3 (NIV)

"For by the grace given me I say to every one of you: Do not think of yourself more highly than you ought, but rather think of yourself with sober judgment, in accordance with the faith God has distributed to each of you."

Romans 12:3 (NIV)

Having Christ as a daily part of our lives allows us to see the perfection of Him in comparison to ourselves. This calls us to strive towards our Heavenly Father and less towards our flawed character. If however, your confidence in who you are is not as high, you may believe most situations are your fault, or you may accept specific behavior because you do not understand that you are worth more and deserve better. Letting God work on your character allows Him to show you what you need to change, all while revealing how amazing you are. God can love and correct at the same time; in fact, that is why He corrects us! He is a friend, Father, encourager, provider, and healer. He can be your source of joy, peace, laughter, truth, and wisdom if you want Him to be. There is a difference however between being insecure and being humble. God calls us into a life that is humble; never forgetting how much we need forgiveness and awareness of our daily mistakes. Staying humble keeps us from becoming proud but also calls us into freedom from our character flaws through life in Christ. We don't have to live insecure about who we are when we have new life in Christ. Let's look at some scriptures that touch on the value of a humble spirit:

"For all those who exalt themselves will be humbled, and those who humble themselves will be exalted."

Luke 14:11 (NIV)

"He guides the humble in what is right and teaches them his way."

Psalms 25:9 (NIV)

"For the LORD takes delight in his people; he crowns the humble with victory."

Psalm 149:4 (NIV)

"For those who exalt themselves will be humbled, and those who humble themselves will be exalted."

Matthew 23:12 (NIV)

Allowing Christ to be at the center of your life before getting into a relationship will show you what you need to change and the love that you deserve. You should not walk through this life over or under-confident, but rather in the grace that God has given you and the acceptance of the fantastic person, He says you are. You can only have this wholeness in yourself through time alone with Christ. God knows exactly who you are now and who He created you to be. Knowing Him means understanding yourself. Having a relationship with the one who knows you best can help you to understand what you struggle with and what you need to change. This helps each of us to identify what we were responsible for in situations and what we were not. Who we are defines how we act, so why not allow God to guide you into the very best version of yourself. It will benefit you to have God's wisdom before trying to bring your flawed opinion into a relationship. No one will benefit from an insecure or prideful individual. Staying humble to your mistakes but aware of the greatness God has given you, helps you to walk with both grace and confidence into any relationship.

Relationships Day 4

Drop Your Mindset and Grab Christ's Character Part 2

Welcome back! Today we are going to be finishing up our topic from yesterday. As you recall, we talked about why it is essential to have a deeply rooted relationship with Christ BEFORE getting into a serious relationship with a significant other. Today we will continue on this topic and talk about another reason why this is absolutely vital:

2. Relationship With Christ Before Your Significant Other Keeps You From Compromising

When you are trying to find the person you want to spend your life with, you have to go into every situation with your foundation in Christ already in place. You have to go into meeting men with a strong commitment to the women of God that you have been called to be. There's a massive difference between merely knowing about God and actually knowing God. When you really know Christ the reasons behind why you do or don't entertain certain situations will have shifted. They've gone past acting out of a sense of obligation or because you've been commanded. Your actions are not based on how guilty you may feel or because you are sinning. When you really know Christ, these feelings are not the motives behind your actions.

For me, I struggled with sexual lusts for years. Thinking about it and engaging in sexual thoughts are just as bad as actually having sex outside of marriage. God says that if you lust after another person, you have already committed adultery in your heart. This type of thinking is not of God and was something that I needed to overcome in my life. Everything changed for me when I began to get closer with God. I was struggling more than I had been in a long time and I was feeling awful about it. I didn't want to keep sinning and thinking these thoughts, but it felt like I had no control. To bring this type of behavior in my next relationship would cause severe problems, so it needed to be fixed beforehand. It was only when I began to get very close to God: reading His Word, listening to sermons and pastors, praying, and just spending quiet time looking to Him, that He revealed the most essential truth about overcoming sin:

You will never be able to uphold the Christian lifestyle especially in your daily relationship with your life partner if you don't have a real understanding of Christ.

Like I said before when you know Christ the reasons behind what you do will be different. Having a grip and a hold on sin before entering a relationship is much easier then if you start off compromising in the relationship. Compromising could be anything: sexual sins, picking up habits that you know are wrong, distancing yourself from church and God because the person you are with does not value it, etc. When you are firmly rooted in Christ before your relationship, you go in knowing your boundaries and what you will and will not tolerate. The Holy Spirit will guide you, and you will be able to tell if the person will lead you closer or farther away from Christ and who you want to be.

Your Life On Earth Needs To Be Centred Around Building Christ-like Character

Every situation, every circumstance, every temptation, every trial; everything you are faced with is an opportunity for you to overcome sin. Sometimes we can be focused on getting into a relationship that we bypass the time that we need to spend with just God working on the character traits we have that will hinder progress in these relationships. Our time here on earth is not about getting married and having kids, yes those can be parts of our lives but they are not the main actions that we should be focused on. Our primary goal on earth is to know Christ and to become more like Him. When becoming more like Christ and developing His character are our top priorities, it allows God to mold us into Christ-centered individuals. The more of Christ we can bring into our relationships, the better. The more Christ-like behavior and character we have, the easier it will be to say no to certain people and choices, and yes to those that bring us closer to Christ. We will no longer make decisions out of insecurities that we have, or an insatiable desire to be loved by someone else. Every action we take will be in alignment with who God says we are and to bring glory to His name. Instead of asking yourself why you haven't been able to find someone or where they are, ask yourself if you are ready to be with them. Don't be so busy trying to find the right person that you neglect becoming that person yourself.

Self Reflection:

- Have you spent time allowing God to work on your character and who you are?
- If you are not in a relationship, are you daily working on your character to become who God called you to be?

- Is the value that you have placed on your partner greater than the amount you have towards your relationship with Christ? How can you adjust this?

Health Check ✓

- Do you encourage your husband/boyfriend to live a healthy life? Do you lead by example?
- If you are single are you creating healthy habits to share in your future relationships?

Takeaways

- Whether single or in a relationship, make God the most important relationship you have. Having Him at the center of your life is the only way you will have lasting, loving relationships
- Don't spend your life searching for a relationship, instead seek God so when you meet that person you will be able to thrive together
- Daily ask God to reveal your character flaws and what you need to work on

Relationships Day 6

What's the Intention Behind Your Actions?

We are going to focus on how we can have healthy friendships in our devotional today. Many relationships in the Bible are examples of Godly friendships, but the one I would like to highlight is between David and Jonathan. There are 3 main attributes this friendship had that we should aim to have in each of ours today.

1. Jonathan and David had a genuine love for each other
To some, this may seem weird, but Jonathan and David's relationship was full of mutual love and respect for each other. When David defeated Goliath, Jonathan was not jealous or envious of this great accomplishment. Rather he admired Davids bravery and courage and expressed that outwardly to him. Many times in our own relationships our insecurities or low self-esteem can stop us from being happy for those that we claim are friends or people we care about. Whether conscious or unconscious, our actions can reflect how we honestly feel and think about ourselves and our friends. With Jonathan and David, there was no underlying reasons, hidden agendas, or envious emotions. Jonathan truly wanted the best for David and vice versa. The Bible says:

"Jonathan made a covenant with David because he loved him as himself. Jonathan took off the robe he was wearing and gave it to David, and with his tunic, and even his sword, his bow, and his belt."

1 Samuel 18:3-4 (NIV)

Mutual love and respect for one another can be hard to find in friendships, especially those with other women. We can feel pitted against one another or give in to feelings of jealousy which can then cause our actions to become tainted with sin. As we continue on with this devotion reflect on your own friendships and how they are.

2. Both Jonathan and David Sacrificed For Each Other

There were many times that Jonathan spoke out against the horrible plans his Father had to kill David. Although Jonathan had not known David that long, his loyalty and love for him urged him to protect him and at many times warn him about the danger that he was in. David also reciprocated this by resisting the urge to go after Jonathan's Father and kill him. There were countless opportunities for David to kill Saul, however out of respect for the covenant that he made with Jonathan and God he did no such thing continuing to show his love and respect for his friend. Sometimes we miss the mark on having our friends back. We may say the wrong words or unintentionally hurt the ones we claim to love. It is not so much about being the perfect friend or getting everything right, but instead about your intentions in your relationships. Jonathan and David's intentions towards each other were pure; meaning all the actions they took towards one another came from the desire to see the very best done in each other's lives. They had a mutual love for one another and therefore protected and respected each other. When we have a low view of who we are it's hard to love our friends from an unbiased perspective. We need to make sure our actions and words are coming from a place of truly wanting and doing what's best for them. These days we hear that you need to look out for yourself first and you need to take care of your needs before you help others. Although there is some truth to that, we also need to understand that true love is a sacrifice. Jesus was the most excellent example of this when He died on the cross for our sins. He took the weight of every sin each of us would commit in our lives and was crucified so that we could live eternally in paradise. It was not convenient, comfortable, or in the best interest of Jesus to die for us. He already lived in eternal paradise with God, but He chose to come to earth to die for us out of love. David and Jonathan understood this concept and in many cases put each other's needs above their own. Because of this, they had a fantastic friendship. The Bible says that "the soul of Jonathan was knit to Davids." The bond and love they had for each other were rare and Godly. The love we have for our friends should reflect the relationship that David and Jonathan had and the love that Jesus shows to us daily. It is essential that we ask ourselves what type of friend we are. Evaluating our patterns in friendships can help us to recognize them when situations arise. Our self-esteem plays a considerable role in how we treat our friends. If we know our actions are coming from a jealous, insecure place, we need to seek God and ask him to help us change this so our relationships will thrive not die!

Self Reflection

- Think of your closest friends right now, how would you describe your relationships with them?
- Do they reflect an unconditional love or are they based on circumstances and what is convenient for you?
- Do you strive to be there and go the extra mile for your friendships?
- Do your friends treat you with reciprocal love and appreciation?
- If not, have you brought it up to them in a loving way? Why or Why not?

Health Check ✓

- Do you encourage your friends to make healthy choices and vice versa? Or do you just allow them to continue in ways that are not beneficial? Why or Why Not?

Takeaways

- Love your friends the way that Jesus loves you! Remind yourself daily of the sacrifice that Jesus made when He died for you.
- Treat your friends how you would want to be treated, not how they always treat you
- Build healthy communication with your friends and express if you do not feel they are treating you with mutual respect and love
- Daily ask yourself if you genuinely want to be friends with the people you have in your life or have they just become space filler relationships

Self Esteem/ Relationships Day 7

Weekly Reflection

Our third week is complete! I hope that this week you were able to learn more about yourself and get closer to our Heavenly Father. I can't wait to share our next and final topics together. Take this time to reflect back on all that we learned by answering the questions below. Ask God to open your eyes and speak to you about what you can take away from this week. Blessings,

Weekly Reflection :

1. What passage and devotion spoke to you the most? Why?
2. What can you take away from this week's topic of possessions and apply to your life starting now?
3. What has God been speaking to you as you read through each passage this week?
4. Before you pray, write out some of your prayer concerns that you need God to help you with in regards to helping shape the person you want to become

Prayer Concerns :

Careers and Equality Intro

We are on the last topic of our four-week journey! I am so happy that you have taken the time to read and reflect on yourself these past few weeks. I hope this devotional has helped push you in the direction of perhaps the beginning, or the continuation of a relationship with your Heavenly Father. Our last topic is all about careers and women's equality. It seemed fitting to put these two topics together because of all the recent discussions surrounding women in the workplace and the injustices that many have experienced there. The first four devotions I touch on a general view of our careers that can be applied to anyone. We will look at where God asks us to place importance in our workplace, but also in our daily activities. Learning about this is a vital tool in helping us to prioritize our lives. As women, we seem to be told what should be of value to us and therefore where we spend our time revolves around those beliefs. Understanding what is actually beneficial to our lives helps us to lean away from the expectations of the world and put more a greater emphasis on God's. The last two devotions are geared towards addressing some of the recurring societal ideas regarding who women should be in and outside of their careers, and looking at it from God's point of view. There are so many beliefs about how women should act, what they should or should not tolerate, what they should be fighting for, and ultimately what they should believe in. Taking on Christ-like behavior helps us to detach from society's standards of who we should be, and follow the only one who knows exactly what is best for us. I think it is so important to reflect an idea rather than just accepting it. The word feminism and the beliefs that go along with it have drastically changed over the years. Breaking down some of the views to understand them better helps us to compare each one to the woman of God we are encouraged to strive towards. Let's continue to learn more about ourselves and better our lives together!

Careers and Equality Day 1

Pursuing Your Passions

I have always been a firm believer in finding and pursuing what you love. I remember when I was in high school and I worked a few after-school jobs. I folded clothes for 8-10 hours, and all I could think about was how unhappy I was. I felt like the world was passing me by and I was stuck in a square refolding the same t-shirts that I had just folded twenty minutes ago. Now don't get me wrong, I know some people that absolutely love working in retail; their good at it and it excites them to go to work. For me, however, this was not the case. I always thought to myself "there has got to be more than this." I carried this mindset with me into university as well and while I was looking for jobs shortly after being done school. I was told by many people to take employment wherever I could find work or just to find something to hold me over. To me, that just didn't make sense. I was not interested in putting one moment of my time or energy into something that did inspire me and that I dreaded going to every day; I didn't want to hate my life because of a paycheque. As I have mentioned earlier, I did not finish university and went to college instead to pursue an entirely different career. So many people told me not to, but it was indeed one of the best decisions I ever made in my life. Discovering my joy and passion for fitness has taught me that it is so important to ask yourself: What do you love? What motivates you? What can you see yourself doing and for the most part enjoying? To many people, this type of thinking does not make sense, but then those are usually the individuals that are driven solely by money or impressing others. If you pursue your passion, you will find yourself. You will find true meaning to your life. It will go far past money or titles because life is more than those things. It is about discovering who God made you to be and then using that to complete the very unique purpose that is on your life. You can only find your true and unique purpose through God. Why? Because He made you! He created you with specific abilities to fulfill a particular mission. Many times we go after jobs or make life choices based off of what we deem is important. Usually what we find essential is based on our families, friends, culture, upbringing, experiences, personal beliefs, or society. When we do this, we take a chance with our lives. We pursue choices that might make us happy; that might be what we are destined to do in this life, and we possibly waste the time we have here. Our real purpose is wrapped up in a relationship with Christ. It is only through knowing God that you can begin to understand yourself. It is absolutely crazy how once you experience and have contact with Christ your mind and thinking shifts. It is no longer about pleasing others but rather discovering the truth from the Creator of everything and everyone. He knows what jobs He has designed you to be incredible at because He gave you exactly what you need to for that task. Every single person has different gifts, don't envy others or take a gamble on your life. Live with purpose! You don't have to walk through life guessing or unhappy. God does not promise that there won't be hard times, but what has gotten me through and continues to, is the security and peace I have in what I know Christ called me to do. I know that as long as I'm listening to Him and following His plan, I am truly living my best-destined life.

Self Reflection

- Don't waste your life trying to be someone else. Ask God to open your eyes about the beautiful women that He has called you to be
- God made you with specific abilities, spend time developing those, not what everyone else is doing
- Make your life about more than a paycheque, find meaning through Christ in where you spend your time
- Life is so much more than just a job! Let God show you where you can be a blessing to yourself and others

Health Check ✓

- What is the reason behind your fitness and health goals? Are they purely aesthetic or are they about more than that? How can you start changing your view on health to be more not exclusively on the physical aspect but also geared towards the mental and spiritual issues as well?
- When it comes to your health goals, do you have unrealistic time frames? Are you able to continue to push through to reach these goals even in moments where it feels as if nothing is being accomplished? What are some ways you can monitor your progress?

Takeaways

- What has been your biggest motivator? Money? Success? Credibility?
- Do you think where you've spent your time and what you value is heavily based around a paycheque? Has this helped you or do you think you could be doing more?
- Have you been asking God what to pursue or going off of what the people around you say to value?

Careers/Equality Day 2

When Your Life Doesn't Look Like Your Promise

Many of us through a relationship with Christ have discovered what we are meant to pursue while here on earth. No one is an accident, so therefore each of us was created with a specific calling. God has slowly revealed to me what I am to pursue while here. He has helped me to discover my passions, talents, and where I able to help others. He has taken my ideas and thoughts and shown me how to create a reality out of them with Him in the center of it all. I sincerely thank God for his constant guidance in my life even when I was not aware of it. He has brought me into the right situations, taken me out of the wrong ones, and showed me how to pursue the best plans as well. Although I live in constant gratefulness to God's wisdom and guidance towards my life, I think we can all have moments of self doubt or discouraging feelings. Sometimes it can feel that you are making little to no progress in your life. Sometimes when we compare the success of those around us and the speed at which they reached it, our lives can appear to be moving in slow motion. I know for myself if I stop and think about everything God has shown me that I will do and can accomplish, I can begin to feel very overwhelmed and full of anxiety. This is not only because it feels too big for me, but also because it appears that nothing is happening in my life. The problem with both of these thoughts is that they are more focused on OUR capabilities and not on his. There are countless individuals in the Bible that encountered angels, prophets, and even God himself, that told them of the many amazing things that they would do or what would happen to them. In almost all of these situations what was promised did not arrive right away. Patience was needed, struggles and temptation were felt, faith was built, and the character needed was to be changed before what God had said came to pass. We live in a culture now where we want everything simultaneously, but let's look at some people in the Bible who built up their patience, trusted God, and received their promises because of it.

Noah

"And the Lord said, "My Spirit shall not contend with humans forever, for they are mortal; their days will be a hundred and twenty years."

Genesis 6:3 (NIV)

God instructed Noah to build an ark 120 years before the flood would even take place. Every single person except for Noah's family laughed, ridiculed, and did not believe him as he warned them to repent and turn to God. To almost everyone, Noah's work and dedication seemed to make little to no sense and hold no reward, but Noah believed God and faithfully prepared the Ark until completion. God told Noah once, and he believed. I am sure it was not easy to be laughed at and treated poorly. I am sure that there were times where Noah may have felt discouraged, but he trusted in the words of God and did not waiver from what he had been called to do.

Abraham

"Abram believed the Lord, and He credited to him as righteousness."

Genesis 15:6 (NIV)

Abraham was promised many things from God: a son of his own, that his heirs would be more than the stars in the sky, and that he would gain possession of an enormous amount of land. God did not give Abraham these promises which then lead to his belief. Instead, the Bible says that Abraham heard what God said, believed, and it was therefore counted to him as righteousness. Can we say that we are like that? Do we understand what God has spoken to us and allow our actions to follow? Or do we lead a life that is heavily reliant on looking at our circumstances; leaving no room for belief in Gods Word? Abraham's faith and trust are what drove him to put action behind his belief by leaving his country and everything that he had to follow God's instruction.

Self Reflection

- Can you hear and serve or do you have to see first before you act?
- Do you need constant reassurance from God or are you willing to step out in faith even when you don't see the big picture?
- Is your trust in God-reliant on having everything right away?

Health Check ✓

- When it comes to your health goals, do you have unrealistic time frames? Are you able to continue to push through to reach these goals even in moments where it feels as if nothing is being accomplished? What are some ways you can monitor your progress?

Takeaways

- Continue after what God has told you to do even if you can't see when it will all come full circle
- Don't be the type of Christian that keeps asking God for signs. If He's given you the direction to go, you can trust that it is the right way to pursue
- Remember that God's timing is perfect. He sits outside of time and space and governs us from above. He knows all and is wiser than any of us. His will is better than ours

Careers/Equality Day 3

Having the Heart of God

One evening I was engaging in my regular bedtime routine with God and was about to begin my prayer. I was feeling slightly discouraged due to feeling a bit lost and confused. I remember saying: "God if you tell me exactly what to do and you speak as clear as I am saying these words right now you know I"ll do it. Not because I don't doubt - I might doubt how it's going to turn out, but I don't doubt if it's right, because I"ll know that the instruction came from you."

God immediately spoke to me and said: "That's your heart. You can go wherever you want because your heart is right."

I felt an overwhelming sense of joy and peace. It's not that God was telling me that I could go out and pursue sinful desires and do whatever I want in that sense. It was more of the understanding that the situation was not as critical as my heart was. I could be in any case or circumstance, and because my heart desires to do what God directs me to do, anything and all things could work out in the best way possible. This is how important our character is to God. He is not looking for those who have everything on paper, he is looking for those with a sincere desire to serve Him with their whole hearts. Let's look at David today, an individual that lived to serve God.

"After removing Saul, he made David their king. God testified concerning him: 'I have found David son of Jesse, a man after my own heart; he will do everything I want him to do."

Acts 13:22 (NIV)

"David served God's purpose in his generation."

Acts 13:36 (NIV)

David was a man that desired to serve God. He valued and respected God's Word and what he told him to do. It was not that David was perfect. He made many mistakes and had to ask for forgiveness on several occasions, it's just that at the root of it all he treasured God's Word and instruction. There was nothing David wasn't willing to do for God. To many people, David would not have been a suitable choice for many reasons. He was small in size and had many older brothers who should have been chosen before him to become king. Yet God used David to kill a giant and chose him as the king because of what others could not see; his heart.

When Samuel came to anoint one of Jesse's sons to become king, he did not know which one it would be. He assumed it would be the eldest, perhaps even the strongest or the biggest but God said:

"Do not consider his appearance or his height, for I have rejected him. The Lord does not look at the things people look at. People look at the outward appearance, but the Lord looks at the heart."

God was able to use David because the desire of his heart reflected Jesus at the Garden of Gethsemane shortly before being crucified.

"Father if you are willing, take this cup from me; yet not my will but yours be done."

Luke 22:42 (NIV)

God used David, not because of his career or title - he was a shepherd, not because of his size or mighty strength - he was the smallest and shortest, and not because of his family - he was the youngest of them all. David was able to be used because his heart desired to do God's will.

Many times in our lives we get it backward. We pursue what seems to make the most "sense" without even a second thought. Our lives can turn into a rolling snowball of ideas and actions; getting bigger and faster with each one we make. One choice leads to another, and before we know it, we have defined our values, purposes, and reason for living on fleeting worldly principles. In many cases, you will find that it is not as essential to make the choices we think are right but rather listen to the voice we know is right.

Self Reflection:

- Many of us want to be used by God in significant ways during our lives, or perhaps God has shown you what you are capable of accomplishing.
- God can only work with those who are willing to listen and obey him even when we don't understand. Can you say this is a daily action in your life?
- In what ways have you been disobeying God or his commandments? Why?
- Name three actions you need to start doing to obey what God has been speaking to you, and name three actions you need to stop that is hindering you from being used by God

Health Check ✓

- Do you listen to the advice provided to you regarding your health or do you eat and live how you prefer?

Takeaways

- Look at your character and your heart before asking God to give you grand careers or positions.
- God can only provide you as much you're ready for
- Daily listen to God's direction and live out what he asks you to do, big or small
- The more you can treasure his voice and guidance, the more you can accomplish

Careers/Equality Day 4

What Life's All About

When you consider the objective of your life what comes to mind? Is it a particular career, or accomplishment that you dream about? There is nothing wrong with having goals and living your life to complete them, in fact, God wants us to do this. As we have gone through each week, I continue to mention that God has a specific plan for each of our lives and with that comes specific goals that he wants us to make a priority. The problem begins when our goals do not line up with God's purposes for our lives. There should be a specific objective or purpose behind every decision we make. Our goals are the actions that we take to accomplish the mission or specific objective. In our last devotion, we talked about how God was able to use David because he desired to serve him. He hated what God hated and loved what God loved. He was passionate about God's Word and following its instruction. Not all of us are called to be pastors or missionaries, but we are called to be disciples; daily living to show others the way to a relationship with Christ. You can serve God whether you are a school teacher or a pilot; the occupation does not matter, but the mindset does. God's purpose needs to be our focus.We are so blessed that we know God! But we are not saved solely to live in grace, we are also called to bring others into this grace through having a relationship with him. When our goals in this life have little to do with the salvation of lost souls and instead are centered around what is best, convenient, or most comfortable, we are not living for the right reasons. Jesus died because of his love for the Father and for us, can we say that we too live with this love for others or are our lives about loving ourselves? Let's read our passage for the day to discover what God says about this:

Reading — Matthew 25: 31-46 (NIV)

The Sheep and the Goats

"When the Son of Man comes in his glory, and all the angels with him, he will sit on his glorious throne. All the nations will be gathered before him, and he will separate the people one from another as a shepherd separates the sheep from the goats. He will put the sheep on his right and the goats on his left.

"Then the King will say to those on his right, 'Come, you who are blessed by my Father; take your inheritance, the kingdom prepared for you since the creation of the world. For I was hungry, and you gave me something to eat, I was thirsty, and you gave me something to drink, I was a stranger, and you invited me in, I needed clothes, and you clothed me, I was sick and you looked after me, I was in prison and you came to visit me.'

"Then the righteous will answer him, 'Lord, when did we see you hungry and feed you, or thirsty and give you something to drink? When did we see you a stranger and invite you in, or needing clothes and clothe you? When did we see you sick or in prison and go to visit you?'

"The King will reply, 'Truly I tell you, whatever you did for one of the least of these brothers and sisters of mine, you did for me.'

"Then he will say to those on his left, 'Depart from me, you who are cursed, into the eternal fire prepared for the devil and his angels. For I was hungry and you gave me nothing to eat, I was thirsty, and you gave me nothing to drink, I was a stranger, and you did not invite me in, I needed clothes, and you did not clothe me, I was sick and in prison and you did not look after me.'

"They also will answer, 'Lord, when did we see you hungry or thirsty or a stranger or needing clothes or sick or in prison, and did not help you?'

"He will reply, 'Truly I tell you, whatever you did not do for one of the least of these, you did not do for me.' "Then they will go away to eternal punishment, but the righteous to eternal life."

Our lives on earth are not our eternity, but they do decide where we will spend it. Everything we do or do not do matters to God. Jesus came here with a clear mission and was faithful until the end. God expects us to continue the mission and lead others into the grace that Jesus gave to us. It is vital that we do not downplay who we are or what God has given us to do. You will stand before God and make an account for where you spent your time. Valuing what the world values may provide you with riches here but it will leave you empty in eternity. Good people and good acts don't secure your salvation or solidify your relationship with Christ. It is only those that confess that Jesus is Lord, live to honor Him with their lives, and bring others into relationship with Him, that will receive eternal life. Our lives can become so diluted when we start to care more about ourselves, money, and jobs, and less about where we and others will spend eternity. Your career may change throughout your lifetime, but your purpose on this earth should never. Your salvation and others should be the main reason for living.

"Not everyone who says to me, 'Lord, Lord,' will enter the kingdom of Heaven,but only the one who does the will of my Father who is in Heaven."

Matthew 7:21 (NIV)

Self Reflection:

- Are our actions about getting closer to what God has told us to accomplish or are we more focused on the goals that the world tells us are important?
- Have we made building relationships with people a priority?
- Think for a moment about what is most important to you? What would be the one thing that you want to accomplish? Is God at the center of it, why or why not?
- How can you make God's plans your plans?

Health Check ✓

- Is your health a priority to you? Do you see the importance of it? Why or Why Not?
- God wants you to bring glory to him not just in your career, but in the way you care for yourself. Do you bring beauty to God with how you treat your physical body? (eating habits, sleep, etc.)

Takeaways

- Ask God how and where he wants you to bring glory to Him. He will always answer and give you the direction that you need

- It's never too late to serve God. No matter who you are and what you've done, there is always a place in the Kingdom of God for you! Find your purpose in Jesus, live in victory, and bring others with you!

Careers and Equality Day 5

Anything You Can Do
I Can Do Better

We are going to transition to our last topic which is Equality. These next 2 devotions will be touching on a few issues regarding the behavior of men and women in and outside of the workplace Understanding ourselves in all four of the subjects that we have reflected upon over the last three weeks is so crucial for us as women. Knowing who we are in Christ and what we can accomplish through Him is vital in becoming the women of God each of us were meant to be. This next devotion will be one topic but broken up into two days. Equality and understanding ourselves is not a subject that I would like to rush by, and want to give us time to dwell in it. As we go through these two devotions, make notes on what touches your heart. Your self-reflection questions will be asked on the second day to sum up both. Let's get started!

In the world today there are many different opinions on gender and equality. The way women are treated in and outside of the workplace and what they should accept from society as a whole has been called into question much more frequently. How men are treated compared to women has been called unfair and unjust. Ideas about what women are capable of (such as a specific position at work) or how men should be allowed to treat them (such as sexual comments and inappropriate language) are being forcefully fought against by many women and in some cases men. There seem to be particular recurring ideas that circulate around these issues:

1. **Women can do anything men can do**
2. **Women should not be treated any differently than a man for engaging in the same behavior, as men are scarcely reprimanded for their actions**
3. **Women or men are more superior than the other (this is believed by both sides for different reasons)**

Before I address these beliefs and apply them to the daily lives of women, let's read our passage today.

Reading — Genesis 2:18-25 (NIV)

The Lord God said, "It is not good for the man to be alone. I will make a helper suitable for him.

Now the Lord God had formed out of the ground all the wild animals and all the birds in the sky. He brought them to the man to see what he would name them; and whatever the man called each living creature, that was its name. So the man gave names to all the livestock, the birds in the sky and all the wild animals.

But for Adam, no suitable helper was found. So the Lord God caused the man to fall into a deep sleep; and while he was sleeping, he took one of the man's ribs and then closed up the place with flesh. Then the Lord God made a woman from the rib he had taken out of the man, and he brought her to the man.

The man said, "This is now bone of my bone and flesh of my flesh; she shall be called 'woman,' for she was taken out of man."

That is why a man leaves his father and mother and is united to his wife, and they become one flesh. Adam and his wife were both naked, and they felt no shame.

From the passage above we can see that God understood then and still sees the need for men and women. Both are important for our world today. Humans as a whole were made in the image and likeness of God, and therefore both have been given equal dignity, but different genders. Why is gender so significant? Well if God believed that man was most effective on his own, he would have stopped creating humans at Adam. As we can see from verse 18 (NIV) God said:

"It is not good for man to be alone; I will make a suitable helper for him."

Another important point to mention is that God could have just made another man for Adam so he could have had a friend and someone to share responsibility with, but God made women instead. God could have continued with the same gender, but He created another with different capabilities and skills to assist Adam. This leads us into our first point mentioned above:

1. Women Can Do Anything Men Can Do

This statement is hazardous for women. It thrives on the notion that men and women are created with the same capabilities and in the exact same way. As we can see in Genesis 2, this just cannot be. If men and women were the same, God would only have needed to create one gender. It is not that women's skills are of lesser value, it is merely that they are different than men. Men and women were meant to complement each other, both work better together and they offer something the other cannot. When we as women are so focused on trying to prove we can do

anything and everything men can do; whether in our workplace or anywhere else in our lives, we miss out on everything we were naturally created to do as a woman. God created two different genders for a reason; everything He does is intentional and for a purpose. Do not try and prove that you are capable, but instead live in the beautiful person God created you to be; as women and as the unique individual that you are. I am sure many of us have experienced times in our lives where we were compared to men.

Our skills and abilities may have been called into question based on the fact that we are women. As we fight towards breaking down these stigmas, I believe it is essential to recognize and understand that we as women are not the same as men, but that in itself is not a negative realization. We complement and fill the gaps with skills they do not have. We are unique, but that does not make us any less equal. Man in himself is limited, flawed, and needs daily character renewing. We should be careful to say that we are just as good as another human being, but instead base our righteousness around Christ; his character and attributes are the only ones that we should strive to be like. Since we have been created to reflect the Creator, we have been filled with worth that goes beyond our gender, social, or economic status and instead rests in the beautiful splendor of our Heavenly Father.

Careers and Equality Day 6

Welcome back! We are going to continue our discussion on Careers and Women by discussing the second point outlined in yesterday's devotion:

2. Women should not be treated any differently than men for engaging in the same behavior, as men are scarcely reprimanded for their actions

There are two questions that we should ask when justifying this point:

- **Is this action, whether done by male or female a sin?**

Living in the idea that we should engage in the activities that men do, inevitably pushes the notion that their behavior is the set standard that we as women should try and live up to or that these actions are okay. This does not just overlap into our careers but in our role as women as a whole and what we bring to the world. The problem we face when making our actions about gender alone is that we miss the most important way we should regulate our choices; this is if it is right or wrong. As Christian women, we know that God is not a respecter of person. Sin is sin, and each of us stands before God to make an account for the way in which we lived our lives. None of us will get a free pass if we happen to be male or if we lived by what the world says is acceptable; this just does not matter.

You stand before God alone, so using the phrase "but they did this or that." will not be a suitable response for your choices. As women, we may feel that we are justified in actions when we see men or others engaging in certain activities. We may have felt limited or degraded in the past and see this type of behavior freeing.

An example of this would be a new age belief that women should not be judged for having various sexual relationships, as men indulge in the same activities and it is seen as acceptable. One set of standards towards men and women that has, and never will change, is God's. If we look at this issues and many others as what it indeed is; disobedience to His Word, rather than a matter of what is acceptable within gender, both male and female would unavoidably be held to the same standard. We as women do not look like men when we engage in certain activities but rather as sinners who have blurred the lines of what is right or wrong by what another group of people has deemed acceptable. Focusing on obeying God's Word rather than gender calls every individual to a higher standard of living.

When Adam and Eve both sinned in the garden of Eden, they were given specific punishments for their crimes. Men's punishment was different than women's, but ultimately they both were sinners and kicked out of the garden of Eden.

Genesis 3:21-24 (NIV)

The Lord God made garments of skin for Adam and his wife and clothed them. And the Lord God said, "The man has now become like one of us, knowing good and evil. He must not be allowed to reach out his hand and take also from the tree of life and eat, and live forever." So the Lord God banished him from the Garden of Eden to work the ground from which he had been taken. After he drove humans out, he placed on the east side of the Garden of Eden cherubim and a flaming sword flashing back and forth to guard the way to the tree of life.

God did exclude Adam or Eve from receiving the consequences for their actions. Focusing on obeying God's Word rather than gender calls every individual to live at a high standard.

- **I can behave how a man does but is it the most effective way?**

Read: 1 Peter 3: 1-5 (NIV)

"Wives, in the same way, submit yourselves to your own husbands so that, if any of them do not believe the word, they may be won over without words by the behavior of their wives, when they see the purity and reverence of your lives.

Your beauty should not come from outward adornment, such as elaborate hairstyles and the wearing of gold jewelry or fine clothes. Rather, it should be that of your inner self, the unfading beauty of a gentle and quiet spirit, which is of great worth in God's sight. For this is the way, the holy women who put their hope in God used to adorn themselves.

Peter is addressing wives in this passage, but this can be applied to women in any role. Here we can see him giving an example of a woman who is a believer in Christ, but her husband is not. The wife, of course, wants her husband to join her in this new found salvation; however he is reluctant, and she doesn't know how to get through to him.

Peter goes on to say that our beauty is seen in our "inner self," and that is in "the unfading beauty of a gentle and quiet spirit." Peter is not implying in these verses that there is something wrong with women who take care of themselves or who put effort into their appearance. Instead, he is saying that woman who rely on physical beauty to strike influence, are much less effective than those inspiring change with who they are. What we as women fail to see is that our power is in our character. The character that Peter is telling women to seek after and embody, influences and inspires much more change in others than anything else. Women lose their impact when they try to enact change either with the wrong element (physical beauty) or in the wrong way (acting like the opposite sex) Many believe taking on the character of men will earn respect but in reality it is when we live in the confidence of being a female that we find our own success. The Bible gives specific instructions to men and women because both have different strengths, weaknesses, and roles. Trying to take on the same attributes of men only diminishes who we are as women and the beauty in that. Nowadays we are told to be just as aggressive and outspoken as men to get the same result, but that is not how God made women. Peter addresses in this passage that if this woman really wants to encourage change in the mind of her husband, that she is not to just say what is right but rather SHOW it through her way of life. Trying to dominate or act like "the head," is counterproductive and ineffective for us women because it is not the way in which we were meant to inspire change. I do not think that we as women should have penalties or privileges stripped from us for acting like men, but I do believe we are doing a disservice to ourselves and the world when we do not live in the specific influence that God gave to women. We would be much better at making a difference if we tried to do it less like males and more in the beauty of being female. Peter references those who have a quiet, gentle spirit and who put their hope in God as "holy women." When our trust, hope, identity, worth, and strength rests in God and who He said we are, we don't need to go around trying to make ourselves known and demand our rights. We walk with confidence, strength, and surety into every circumstance and situation because we know that God has justified us and even if others cannot see our worth and value, He does. He will always provide justice and protection to the woman that follows after holiness before trying to prove themselves to others.

Self Reflection

- Do you base your daily actions around what is accepted by society or how God says we as women should behave?
- Have you become hyper-focused on proving your capabilities to others? If so, why?
- Do you work at developing the natural character traits that God has given you as a woman or are you more focused on living the way others do?

Health Check ✓

- Are the standards of care to your physical body (what you eat, sleep patterns, physical fitness) based off of the people around you, or is it based off how Christ tells us to care for it?

Takeaways

- Focus your attention on who God says you are, not on who others say you arent or who they want you to be!
- Don't live your life trying to prove your worth or talent, follow after Christ and no one can stand in your way.
- Live building holy character, not pursuing sinful actions no matter what gender is engaging in them

Careers and Equality Day 7
Weekly Reflection

We have come to the end of our four-week journey together. I pray that you have been able to take even one day, passage, scripture, or lesson and apply it to your life. My prayer is that you were able to continue to grow your faith and grow with God each day. Take the time to reflect below on the entire month and what you were able to take away from it. Thank you for letting me be a part of your spiritual journey. Blessings,

Yvonne

Printed in the United States
By Bookmasters